Oral Diag
the Clinician's
Guide

Warren Birnbaum BDS FDS RCS
Associate Specialist/Consultant
and Head of the Department of Primary Dental Care

and

Stephen M. Dunne BDS FDS RCS PhD
Senior Lecturer/Honorary Consultant,
Department of Conservative Dentistry

The Guy's, King's and St Thomas' Dental Institute,
King's College, London, UK

wright

OXFORD AUCKLAND BOSTON JOHANNESBURG MELBOURNE NEW DELHI

Wright
An imprint of Elsevier Science Limited
Robert Stevenson House,
1–3 Baxter's Place, Leith Walk,
Edinburgh EH1 3AF

First published 2000
Reprinted 2002

British Library Cataloguing in Publication Data
A catalog record for this book is available from the British Library

Library of Congress Cataloging in Publication Data
A catalog record for this book is available from the Library of Congress

ISBN 0 7236 1040 1

Composition by Scribe Design, Gillingham, Kent
Printed and bound by MPG Books Ltd, Bodmin, Cornwall

Contents

Preface

The foundation of any form of successful treatment is accurate diagnosis. Though scientifically based, dentistry is also an art. This is evident in the provision of operative dental care and also in the diagnosis of oral and dental diseases. While diagnostic skills will be developed and enhanced by experience, it is essential that every prospective dentist is taught how to develop a structured and comprehensive approach to oral diagnosis. Our objective is to contribute to and facilitate this process.

We have carefully selected the title of this book in an attempt to reflect the authors' aims and the contents. The book is written by clinicians for clinicians to provide a structured guide to the novice and a source of revision for the more experienced. It is intended primarily for undergraduate dental students and newly qualified practitioners. The authors acknowledge the enormous contribution made by our current and recent students with their feedback and advice on the development of the text such that it would be truly useful to them; indeed even the format of the text, in particular the frequent use of bullet points, is as they requested.

Our original aim was to produce a slim, pocket-sized book that could be carried on clinic but as with most books of this nature, being brief meant omitting information our students considered essential. Thus the book is larger than was originally anticipated but we hope with good reason. Despite this the book cannot cover everything! Most chapters can be or have been the subject of a complete textbook in their own right. Instead it is intended to be used as an adjunct to clinical teaching and standard texts, not as a total replacement. After most of the chapters we have suggested further reading for those wanting to delve into specific conditions further.

We have endeavoured to guide the reader through the history, examination and diagnostic tests necessary to establish a diagnosis. We have included advice and notes based on the authors' experience that we hope will prove helpful to the new clinician.

Chapters 5 and 6 consider pain of dental and non-dental origin relating to the head and neck. We hope that the reader will consider the emphasis given to this important subject is appropriate. Subsequent chapters consider trauma, infection, cysts, ulcers, white patches, bumps, lumps and swellings, oral changes in systemic disease and oral consequences of medication. Where appropriate, chapters include a differential diagnosis which we trust may also assist the student in revision for their professional examinations. Additional details relating to the history, examination and diagnostic tests, particularly relevant to the subject of each chapters, are also included. Readers are advised to consult textbooks on histology for detailed descriptions of these lesions referred to in the text. Attempting to include histological details would have made the book far too large and was contrary to the advice of our students. Similarly, in many cases treatment options have not been included and the reader is referred to other texts on the subjects, some of which are listed at the end of the relevant chapters.

We do appreciate that acquiring diagnostic skills requires practice, experience and even a degree of intuition. However, we hope that the student who follows the guidance and recommendations in this book will find it a stimulating and interesting learning curve rather than a traumatic experience for both themselves and their patients.

Acknowledgements

We are greatly indebted to our current and recent students for their advice and enthusiasm as the text evolved to create a textbook they would wish to use themselves. We are also grateful to Malcolm Bishop, Dr Caroline Pankhurst and particularly to Professor Stephen Porter for their invaluable advice, suggestions and for reading the initial drafts.

We would also like to thank Mrs Margaret Piddington and Mrs Lucinda Dunne for their secretarial and administrative support. We are indebted to Mr Eric Whaites and Mrs Jan Farthing of the Department of Dental Radiology, Guy's, King's and St Thomas' Dental Institute, Denmark Hill Campus, for the loan of radiographs which have been used to illustrate Chapter 12.

We acknowledge the help of Mary Seager, Claire Hutchins and Hannah Jones, from our publishers Butterworth-Heinemann, for their advice, support and continuous encouragement. Finally we would like to thank our families for their forbearance during the writing of this text.

1

The challenge of diagnosis

Oral diagnosis, like diagnosis of disease in other parts of the body, is complicated by many factors:

- Symptoms of quite different diseases may be similar; in some cases exactly similar, e.g. pulpitis and atypical odontalgia (see Chapter 5). ***A symptom is defined as any bodily change perceptible to the patient.***
- Signs of different diseases may be similar. An ulcer, for example, may be caused by minor trauma from a sharp tooth or potentially be a squamous cell carcinoma. ***A sign is defined as any bodily change which is perceptible to a trained observer.***
- Signs and symptoms of the same disease, suffered by different patients, may be very different. For example, an excruciating pain described by one may be perceived as discomfort by another.
- Signs and symptoms may be hidden. It is the dentist's task, by careful questioning and observation to render these 'visible'.
- Preconceived ideas may cloud the perspective of the patient, who may have decided that the problem is 'dental' and has, therefore, sought the advice of a dentist. In this way they may fail to reveal appropriate details to the dentist and non-dental causes of oral problems may be missed, despite repeated and adequate questions.

- Common disease (e.g. pulpitis) occurs frequently and must be excluded before the rarity is considered. However, the rarity will occasionally present, and hence the dentist must learn to expect the unexpected.
- Some patients may provide the history that they believe the dentist wants to hear, and which is socially acceptable. For example, patients may underestimate their alcohol, tobacco and sugar consumption while the time spent on tooth cleaning may be overestimated. In addition, a history of misuse of drugs, sexually transmitted diseases, eating disorders or child abuse may not readily be admitted to a dentist.
- Relevant but non-dental matters, for example the medical history, may erroneously be considered, by some patients, to be none of a dentist's business!
- While the process of diagnosis, quite rightly, begins as soon as a patient enters the surgery, appearances can be deceptive. A smart suit, for example, does not confer immunity to high alcohol and tobacco use, or dental neglect.

The system of diagnosis of disease involves three main elements:

1. History
2. Examination
3. Diagnostic tests

General considerations:

- Patients should be respectfully treated as an individual, not as a disease requiring treatment.
- Always use a methodical approach, avoiding 'spot' diagnoses.

While the experienced clinician will appear to diagnose a problem with minimal attention to peripheral details, this technique may lead the inexperienced clinician to guess-work. Experience is gained by practice in the consideration of all details. Only with experience is it possible to reject those enquiries and investigations irrelevant to the particular patient under consideration.

- The dental record contains important facts. Neither hide such facts amongst irrelevant detail nor omit them.
- The dental record should be dated, complete, legible and indelible and signed by the clinician. The record may be required by other clinicians and occasionally by members of the legal profession.
- The patient has a legal right to access their dental record: do not enter any disparaging remarks.

- During a clinical consultation a third person, such as the dental nurse, should be present at all times. This chaperone should not be a lay person since emergency procedures may need to be followed and equipment operated.
- The consent of a parent/legal guardian is required for children under 16 years old.
- Children are often more cooperative and communicative if, after the initial introduction, the accompanying parent is asked to return to the waiting area.
- Establishing rapport with the patient is an essential prerequisite for obtaining an adequate history.

Establishing rapport

The initial patient interview consists of an exchange of both verbal and non-verbal information. The dentist's posture and demeanour can do much to enhance or ruin rapport:

- The patient should be at the same eye level as the clinician; not lying flat.
- Make eye contact, but do not stare as this may be intimidating.
- The patient should be reasonably close to the clinician, approximately one metre away. Proximity denotes intimacy, whereas excess distance suggests inattentiveness.
- A forward lean towards the patient promotes the impression of attentiveness.
- Likewise, facing the patient indicates attentiveness, while turning away suggests rejection.
- A smile or confirmative nod of the head shows warmth and concern.
- Record details of the patient's close family and any forthcoming social events (e.g. marriages, births) that may be volunteered. Reference to these, subsequently, establishes personal rapport.
- The initial interview should be conducted free of any protective eyewear and mask, otherwise, facial expressions are concealed and speech is muffled. Protective wear should be placed only when the physical examination begins.
- Before any investigation or procedure, tell the patient what you will be doing and when and why you will be doing it. A patient surprised by any action may become frightened, leading to a possible loss of trust.

Conclusion

A relaxed patient, an attentive, thorough and methodical dentist, in a friendly but professional environment are the foundations of oral diagnosis.

The history

'Listen to your patient, he is telling you the diagnosis!'
(Dia-gnosis: [Greek] through knowledge)

Summary

1. **Introductory phase**
   Greetings
   Patient's initial statement
   Biograpical data
2. **Listening to the patient's account**
   Present complaint (CO)
3. **Structured questioning**
   History of present complaint (HPC)
   Medical history (MH)
   Dental history (DH)
   Family history (FH)
   Social history (SH)

Objectives

- To establish rapport between patient and dentist.
- To gather sufficient information to arrive at a provisional diagnosis.
- To gain an understanding of the patient's wishes and expectations.

The history

- Is a personal account of the patient's problem.
- Is often the most important component of clinical diagnosis.
- May occasionally be the only diagnostic factor (cf. pain. See Chapters 5 and 6).
- Some patients (e.g. young children or those with special needs) may be unable to provide an accurate history. If this is the case,

in extreme circumstances, questions may be addressed to a parent/guardian/carer. However, it is usually better to persevere with the patient, even if this means asking leading questions, since it is they who are suffering the problem. A third party may apply yet another interpretation of the problem.
- With extreme language difficulties, encourage the patient to bring an interpreter. Here again, it is better to persist with the patient, wherever possible, although this is clearly often difficult.

The history includes three main stages:
1. A brief introductory phase.
2. Listening to the patient's account.
3. Structured questioning.

Stage 1. The introductory phase
- Greet the patient by name.
- Introduce yourself by name and describe your role in helping the patient.
- 'Break the ice' by greeting with an introductory comment about the weather, the patient's journey or occupation, or a compliment (but avoid excessive flattery).
- Most patients do not understand medical/dental terminology; use plain speech but do not 'talk down'. A useful 'rule of thumb' is to employ only vocabulary that might be found in a popular newspaper.
- Record the patient's initial statement. This may, or may not, relate to their reason for attendance but may often provide important information. The statement, 'I'm terrified of dentists but the pain forced me here' has obvious implications for the patient's management.
- Record or check biographical data, including:

Patient's name

Gender

Date of birth (cf. age-related diseases: most patients with oral cancer are over 40 years old)

Address (difficulty in attendance, fluoridation of local water supply)

Telephone number—daytime and residential

Occupation (education, socio-economic status, exposure to sunlight—skin and lip cancer, chef—caries)

Names and addresses of general medical practitioner and general dental practitioner

Stage 2. Listening to the patient's account

The present complaint (CO, Complains Of):

This is the reason the patient is seeking care.
- Use an opening question, such as 'How can I help you?'
- If a list of problems is forthcoming, ask 'What is your main concern?'

Notes:
- Encourage the patient to describe their problem.
- In general, do not interrupt the patient.
- Encourage the inarticulate by simple questioning.
- Direct the 'talkative' to more relevant matters.
- Record the complaint in the patient's own words. Particularly in medicolegal cases, the patient's words may be set in inverted commas.
- In describing the present complaint, the patient is listing symptoms (see Chapter 1).
- Record symptoms in order of severity.
- If you cannot interpret an adjective describing a symptom it is often useful to ask the patient for a word that describes the opposite to it.
- Relate the present complaint to the initial statement made by the patient.

Stage 3. Structured questioning

This is subdivided into five headings:
1. History of the present complaint.
2. Medical history.
3. Previous dental history.
4. Family history.
5. Social history.

- Open-ended questions, that do not have simple yes or no answers, allow patients more latitude to express themselves.

1. History of the present complaint (HPC)
- Is a chronological account of the development of the problem.
- Include the following questions:

When did you first notice the problem?
How has it changed since? Is it getting worse, better, or staying the same?

Did (or does) anything cause the problem or make it worse? (e.g. heat, cold or eating may aggravate toothache).
Does anything relieve the problem? (e.g. non-prescription analgesics might relieve mild to moderately severe dental pain).

- Proceed through questions relating to any additional symptoms and the effectiveness, or otherwise, of any previous treatments.
- Symptoms may require further clarification. Pain is a subjective symptom and unlike an ulcer, there may be nothing to assess visually. The history is, therefore, of paramount importance (see Chapters 5 and 6).
- Avoid 'leading' questions; suggestible patients may agree to symptoms they did not know they had. Thus, do not ask 'Do you experience pain with hot and cold foods?' Instead, ask 'What causes the pain to start?'
- If 'leading' questions are unavoidable, allow a range of possibilities from which the patient may select.

A complaint of ulceration (see Chapter 10)

A complaint of swelling (see Chapter 12)

2. Medical history (Abbreviated MH)

- May provide important clues to the diagnosis.
- May greatly modify any treatment plan.
- An inadequate medical history may put the health of the patient, the dentist and support staff at risk.
- Is mandatory for medicolegal reasons.
- If a self-administered medical history questionnaire is used, answers must be followed up by the dentist.
- The following questions should be asked:

Have you ever had a serious illness or been in hospital? (Hospitalization often indicates a serious problem).
Have you ever had an operation? (May indicate a serious problem or detail information of the patient's tolerance of an anaesthetic).
If so, did you have any problems? (Excessive bleeding, drug reactions, etc.).
Are you presently under the care of a doctor? (May indicate a serious problem).
Are you taking any tablets, medicines, pills, drugs or creams? (May suggest the underlying problem. Also, drugs prescribed for dental problems may interact with existing medication. Broad spectrum antibiotics may reduce the effectiveness of oral contraceptives, for example, and a barrier method of contraception should be advised).

Have you ever had excessive bleeding after cuts or tooth extraction? (May indicate bleeding tendency).
Have you ever been turned down as a blood donor? (Blood-borne viruses etc).
Have you ever had jaundice, hepatitis or any liver problem? (Risk of cross-infection, delayed drug metabolism, bleeding problem).
Do you have any heart problems? (Risk of angina/heart attack, general anaesthetic risk).
Have you ever had rheumatic fever, a heart murmur, or heart valve problems? (Risk of infective endocarditis following dental procedures).
Have you ever had high blood pressure? (Risk of stroke or cardiac arrest).
Do you have asthma or any chest or breathing problems? (General anaesthetic risk).
Have you ever had tuberculosis? (Risk of cross infection).
Have you ever had any other infectious diseases? (Risk of cross infection).
Are you diabetic? (More susceptible to infection, periodontal disease, risk of collapse if blood sugar falls, general anaesthetic risk).
Have you ever had epilepsy? (Risk of seizure).
Are you pregnant or a nursing mother? (Females only!).
Do you have any allergies, e.g. hay fever, asthma, eczema or to elastoplast? (Adverse reaction to drugs, general anaesthetic risk).
Have you had any problems with antibiotics, particularly penicillin? (Risk of allergic reaction including anaphylactic shock).
Have you had any problems with any tablets or medicines, e.g. aspirin? (Adverse drug reaction).
Have you had any problems with dental or general anaesthetics? (Adverse drug reaction).
Is there any other medical information that I should know? (General 'catch all').

- Check the medical history at each recall appointment; it may have altered significantly in the interim (e.g. anticoagulants, heart attack etc.).
- Contact the patient's doctor/attending physician or surgeon if in doubt.
- If the patient is uncertain of the name or type of any medication, ask them to bring the medication to the next appointment.
- A medical examination may be required for patients under-

going general anaesthesia or sedation and patients with a positive history about to undergo extensive treatment under local anaesthesia.

3. Previous dental history (DH)

- Ask the following questions:

  How often did you visit your previous dentist? (Motivation, likely future attendance).

  When did you last see your dentist and what did your dentist do? (May hint at the present problem).

  Have you ever had orthodontic treatment? (May indicate good motivation).

  Have you ever had any problems with previous treatment/anaesthesia? (Anxiety, health problem).

  How often do you brush your teeth and for how long. Do you use dental floss, or fluoride? (Motivation, knowledge of prevention).

4. Family history (FH)

- If a diagnosis involving a hereditary condition is suspected, include details of the health, age and medical history of parents, grandparents, siblings and children.
- Some diseases, such as haemophilia are notably hereditary, while in others a hereditary disposition may be present, including:

  Non-insulin dependent diabetes mellitus
  Hypertension
  Some types of epilepsy
  Heart disease
  Some psychiatric conditions
  Breast cancer
  Some other malignancies

5. Social history (SH)

- The object is to obtain a profile of the patient's lifestyle which may exert a major influence on the patient's dental and general health.
- Include details of:

  Exercise (anaesthetic risk).
  Body weight relative to height (eating disorders).
  Diet (vegetarian, high acid content, cariogenicity etc.).
  Alcohol consumption (periodontal disease, acute necrotizing ulcerative gingivitis (ANUG), oral cancer, liver cirrhosis, bleeding risk).

Tobacco smoking (periodontal disease, anaesthetic risk, ANUG, oral cancer). Alcohol and cigarette smoking together greatly increase the risk of oral cancer.
Tobacco and betel quid chewing (oral cancer).
Home conditions/partner (neglect, stress).
Residence abroad (tropical diseases).
Work (physical/psychological stress).
Stress (psychosomatic disorders).
Use of non-prescription ('recreational') drugs (cross-infection risk, dental neglect, cardiac risks with cocaine, caries risk with methadone).

Conclusions

The history will often suggest a provisional diagnosis or at the least, the history will allow a differential diagnosis.

The provisional or differential diagnosis will be confirmed or rejected by clinical examination and diagnostic tests.

3

Examination

Summary

1. **General observation**
2. **Extraoral examination (EO)**
   Head, face, neck
   Eyes
   Lips
   Lymph nodes
   Salivary glands
   Temporomandibular joints
   Masticatory muscles
3. **Intraoral examination (IO)**
   Lining mucosa
   Tongue
   Floor of mouth
   Hard and soft palate
   Throat
   Salivary glands
   Salivary flow
   Periodontium
   Teeth
   Referral to a specialist

Clinical examination consists of three main stages:

1. Observation of the patient's general health and appearance.
2. Extraoral examination of the head and neck.
3. Examination of the intraoral tissues.

- Observation begins as soon as the patient enters the surgery.
- During the examination the clinician elicits signs (see Chapter 1).
- Like the history, the examination must be thorough and methodical.

Stage 1. General observation

- Note problems such as:

Body weight, fit of clothes (recent weight loss may indicate serious underlying pathology, e.g. cancer. Very low body weight may suggest an eating disorder. Excessive weight may suggest risk of heart attack or stroke, particularly with a general anaesthetic).

Breathlessness after minor exertion (may indicate heart or lung disorder).

Physical disability.

Obvious illness.

Apparent age, relative to chronological age.

Complexion (pallor with anaemia, yellow with jaundice).

Exposed skin areas, including head, neck, hands and nails (any obvious lesion which may be visible, e.g. finger clubbing).

Facial scarring (previous surgery, trauma, fights).

Stage 2. Extraoral examination (EO)

Head, face and neck
Eyes
Lips
Lymph nodes
Salivary glands
Temporomandibular joint
Masticatory muscles

1. Head, face and neck

Visually examine the face and neck from the front. Look for obvious lumps, defects, skin blemishes, moles, gross facial asymmetry (most faces are slightly asymmetric) or facial palsy (see also pages 105–107).

To visually examine the neck, ask the patient to tilt the head back slightly to extend the neck. Any swelling or other abnormality is clearly seen in this position. Watch the patient swallow; thyroid swellings move on swallowing.

The patient should then turn the head, still with the neck extended, first to the left and then to the right, to allow visual examination of the submandibular region on each side. Except in the most obese, swellings of the sublingual glands, the lymph nodes and the submandibular glands will be seen.

The neck should then be relaxed to allow bilateral examination of the region of the parotid glands.

Note: Unilateral swelling of the parotid salivary glands suggests:

Obstruction of the duct
Tumour
Abscess
Retrograde infection of the gland

Bilateral swelling of the parotid salivary gland suggests:

Viral infection, e.g. mumps
Degenerative changes, e.g. sialosis

2. Eyes (if history suggests)

Look for:

Blinking rate (low frequency staring might indicate a psychological problem, or possibly Parkinson's disease. High frequency may indicate anxiety or dryness of the eyes, e.g. Sjögren's syndrome).

Limitation of ocular movement or strabismus (fractured zygoma).

Exophthalmos (tumour of orbit or cavernous sinus thrombosis).

Bilateral exophthalmos (hyperthyroidism — Graves' disease).

Subconjunctival haemorrhage (fractured zygoma or nasal arch).

Ulceration of conjunctiva (Behçet's disease, mucous membrane pemphigoid).

Conjunctival pallor (anaemia).

Blue sclera (rarely osteogenesis imperfecta).

Yellow sclera (jaundice).

Corneal scarring (mucous membrane pemphigoid).

Dry eyes, conjunctivitis (Sjögren's syndrome).

3. Lips

Visual examination: Note muscle tone (e.g. drooping of the commissure and inability to purse the lips with Bell's palsy), any changes in colour or texture, ulceration, patches, herpetic lesions, angular cheilitis. Note also lip competency/incompetency.

Bimanual palpation: Palpate for lumps, using thumb and forefinger, one intraoral and the other extraoral.

4. Lymph nodes

(See also Chapter 12)

Important — A normal lymph node cannot be felt. If a node is palpable it must be abnormal.

Lymph node anatomy (Fig. 3.1)
The lymph nodes of the head and neck are divided into two main groups:

A. Circular groups
B. Cervical groups

A. Circular groups (arranged around base of skull)
These are sub-divided into outer and inner circular groups:

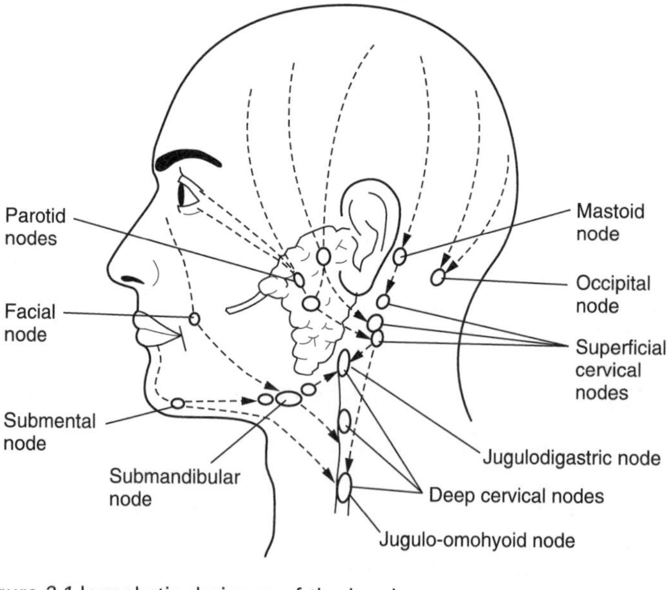

Figure 3.1 Lymphatic drainage of the head.

Outer circle:

Submental — behind the chin, lying on the mylohyoid muscle.
Submandibular — between the mandible and the submandibular salivary gland.
Facial (buccal) — on the buccinator muscle, anterior to the insertion of the masseter muscle.
Mastoid (post-auricular) — on the mastoid process.
Parotid (pre-auricular) — in front of the tragus of the ear.
Occipital — around the occipital artery.

Inner circle (not illustrated in Fig. 3.1). Named nodes include:

Retropharyngeal
Pre-tracheal
Para-tracheal

The circular groups drain into the deep cervical chain.

2. Cervical groups

Superficial cervical nodes (distributed around the external and anterior jugular veins). These drain into the deep cervical chain.

Deep cervical chain (distributed along the internal jugular vein). Important named nodes include:

Jugulodigastric (between the angle of the mandible and the anterior border of the sternomastoid muscle).

Jugulo-omohyoid (just behind the internal jugular vein, above the inferior belly of omohyoid, under cover of the posterior border of sternomastoid).

Drainage (see Fig. 3.1)

Submandibular nodes (unilateral drainage):

These drain the centre of the forehead, frontal and maxillary sinuses, upper lip, external nose, related cheek, upper and lower teeth and gums, anterior two-thirds of the tongue (except the tip) and floor of the mouth. The submandibular node, in turn, drains into the jugulo-omohyoid and jugulodigastric nodes.

Facial (buccal) nodes:

Drain part of the cheek and lower eye lid. The facial node drains into the deep cervical chain.

Parotid (pre-auricular) nodes:

Drain the forehead, temple, vertex, eye lids and orbit. The parotid nodes drain into the superficial cervical and deep cervical chain.

Occipital and mastoid (post-auricular):

Drain the scalp.

Retropharyngeal nodes:
Drain the soft palate and drain into the deep cervical chain.
Submental nodes (drain bilaterally):
Drain the tip of the tongue, lower lip, chin and incisor teeth and gum area. The submental nodes drain to the submandibular nodes or directly into the jugulo-omohyoid node.
Jugulo-omohyoid nodes:
Drain the posterior third of the tongue.

Clinical examination of the lymph nodes

Most lymph nodes should be examined by extraoral, bimanual, palpation from behind the patient:

Expose the neck by asking the patient to loosen relevant clothing. Do not extend the neck since sternomastoid must be relaxed. Use the pulp of the finger tips and try to roll the gland against adjacent harder structures.

Submental — Tip the head forward and try to roll the node against the inner aspect of the mandible.

Submandibular — Same as above but with the patients head tipped to the side being examined (Fig. 3.2).

Jugulodigastric — Move the anterior border of sternomastoid back.

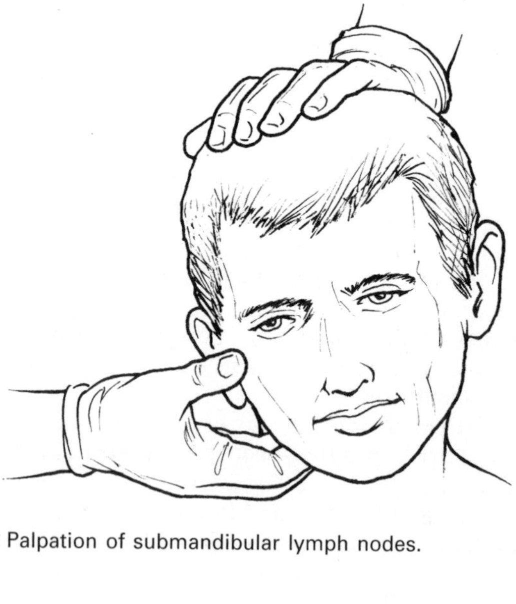

Figure 3.2 Palpation of submandibular lymph nodes.

Jugulo-omohyoid — Move the posterior border of sternomastoid forward.

If a node is palpable, record the:

Site.

Size (measure using vernier callipers).

Texture — soft (infective), rubbery hard (possible Hodgkin's), stony hard (secondary carcinoma).

Tenderness to palpation (infection).

Fixation to surrounding tissues (may suggest metastatic cancer).

Coalescence (e.g. tuberculosis).

Number of nodes (multiple — glandular fever, leukaemia, etc.). If more than one node is found, refer for examination of the rest of the body for generalized lymphadenopathy and blood tests.

Palpable node charactistics:

Acute infection — large, soft, painful, mobile, discrete, rapid onset.

Chronic infection — large, firm, less tender, mobile.

Lymphoma — rubbery hard, matted, painless, multiple.

Metastatic cancer — stony hard, fixed to underlying tissues, painless.

If a non-dental cause is suspected, refer urgently for medical assessment. Suspect metastatic cancer or lymphoma until proven otherwise.

5. Salivary glands

i. Parotid salivary gland
View from the front. The lower part of the ear lobe may be turned outward if the gland is swollen. Palpate the glands for enlargement or tenderness. The gland is located mainly distal to the ascending ramus of the mandible. Occasionally a better view of the parotid gland may be obtained from the back of the patient.

ii. Submandibular salivary gland
Bimanual palpation (Fig. 3.3): Use index and middle finger of one hand intraorally and the same fingers of the other hand extraorally. Palpate the gland above and below mylohyoid and do not neglect to examine the ducts of the glands for calculi.

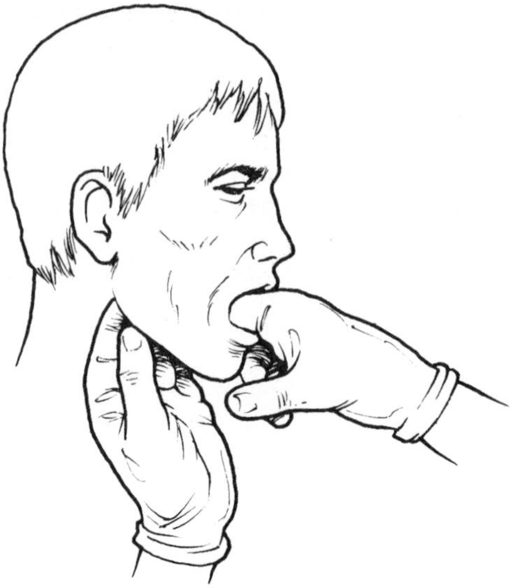

Figure 3.3 Bimanual palpation of the submandibular gland.

6. Examination of articulatory system (if history indicates)

i. Temporomandibular joints (TMJ)

Investigate the following:

Range of movement
Tenderness
Sounds
Locking
Muscle tenderness
Bruxism
Head/neck ache
Occlusion

Range of movement

Measure the maximum pain-free jaw opening, then measure the maximum opening possible, at the central incisor tips. Identify whether limitation is caused by pain or physical obstruction. Observe any lateral deviation.

Notes:

- Any lateral deviation on opening is usually towards the affected (e.g. painful) side.

- The lower limit for normal maximum inter-incisal opening is 35 mm (female), 40 mm (male) (approximately two patient finger-widths).
- Measurement in millimetres, using a rule or calliper, is preferable to measurement of mouth opening in terms of the number of the patient's fingers that can be inserted.
- Trismus is the inability to open the mouth (see below).

Next, measure the extent of lateral excursion, both pain-free and forced. Measure from the centre lines.

Notes:
- The lower limit for normal lateral excursion is 8 mm, in either direction.
- If the left TMJ is painful, the right lateral excursion is usually reduced.
- Mandibular movement may be limited by:
  Trauma, e.g. third molar surgery, local anaesthetic injection, fracture of mandible, middle third of face or zygomatic arch, laceration of masticatory muscles.
  Infection, e.g. pericoronitis, submasseteric, pterygomandibular, infratemporal or parapharyngeal space infections, tonsillitis, mumps, osteomyelitis.
  Scar tissue formation, e.g. post-irradiation, burns, submucous fibrosis, scleroderma.
  Temporomandibular joint disorders (see pages 116–119)
  Central nervous system disorders, e.g. tetanus, meningitis, Parkinson's disease.
  Medication/ poisons, e.g. phenothiazine group of drugs, strychnine.
  Neoplasm, e.g. nasopharyngeal carcinoma (see page 116), coronoid hyperplasia.
  Psychological, e.g. hysteria.

TMJ Tenderness
Use bimanual palpation by pressing over the lateral aspect of the joint. Follow this by intra-auricular palpation by placing the little fingers into the external auditory meatus and gently pressing forwards (Fig. 3.4).

TMJ Sounds
Clicks are caused by sudden movement of the disc relative to the condyle. Clicks may be early (i.e. in the early part of jaw opening), late (may indicate greater disk displacement and are often

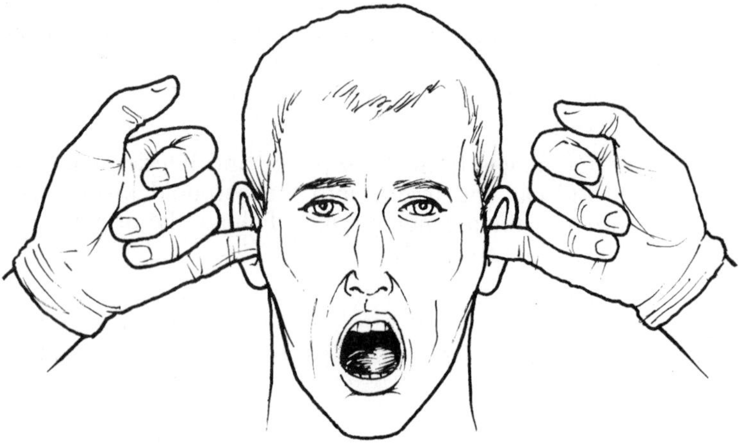

Figure 3.4 Intra-aural palpation of temporomandibular joints.

louder), reciprocal (on opening and closing), single (usual), multiple (unstable or perforated disk), loud, soft, painful or not, and may occur with crepitus (see below).

Fifty per cent of the population experience clicking during their life. It is usually of limited duration and if not causing problems should remain untreated!

Crepitus is a prolonged, continuous, grating or crackling noise. Crepitus occurs with degenerative diseases and acute inflammation (e.g. after trauma).

TMJ Locking

Locking is due to malposition and distortion of the disc, which allows the condyle to rotate but not translate. The jaw may open up to 20 mm and then 'stick'. Rarely, the jaw may open but fail to close easily.

Dislocation

The condyle is displaced over the articular eminence. This may be caused by trauma (e.g. following a difficult tooth extraction) or, very rarely, on yawning.

ii. Muscles of mastication

Examine for tenderness:

Muscles should be tested where they attach to bone. The body of a muscle is not usually tender.

Masseter: Originates from the anterior two-thirds of the zygomatic arch and inserts into the outer aspect of the angle of the mandible. Use bimanual palpation, with the finger of one hand intraoral, index and mid finger of the other hand on the cheek. Palpate the origin and insertion.

Temporalis: Originates from the superior and inferior temporal lines above the ear and inserts into the coronoid process and anterior border of the ascending ramus. Palpate the origin extra-orally and insertion intraorally.

Lateral pterygoid: Originates from the lateral surface of the lateral pterygoid plate and inserts into the anterior border of the condyle and disk. It is inaccessible to palpation. Attempts to palpate behind the maxillary tuberosity are unreliable. Resistance provided by the operator's hand to attempted lateral excursion by the patient may elicit lateral pterygoid pain, and is a more reliable guide.

Medial pterygoid: Originates between the medial and lateral pterygoid plates and inserts into the medial surface of the angle of the mandible. It is not accessible to comfortable palpation.

Occasionally, a more extensive examination may include the sternomastoid, trapezius, and digastric muscles.

Stage 3. Intraoral examination (IO)

- A systematic approach must be adopted to ensure that all areas are examined. Few patients have died as a result of dental caries but many have died as a result of the late diagnosis of oral cancer. Dentists have a duty to detect both potentially malignant and malignant oral lesions.

Examine
Lining mucosa
Tongue
Floor of mouth and ventral surface of tongue
Hard and soft palate
Throat
Salivary glands
Salivary flow
Periodontium
Teeth

Method
- Remove any dentures.
- Use gloved fingers or, when access is very limited, two mouth mirrors, to retract the tissues.
- Use visual inspection supplemented by palpation of any suspicious lesions.

Lining mucosa

Terminology used to describe mucosal lesions:

Erosion — Partial loss of surface epithelium without exposure of underlying connective tissue.

Ulcer — Full thickness loss of surface epithelium with exposure of underlying connective tissue (see Chapter 10).

Vesicle — Circumscribed accumulation of fluid within or below epithelium, less than 5 mm in diameter.

Bulla — Circumscribed accumulation of fluid within or below epithelium, larger than 5 mm in diameter.

(*Note:* Intraorally, vesicles and bullae are often found in a burst condition, appearing as ulcers).

Plaque — Large circumscribed elevated area.

Papule — Small circumscribed elevated area.

Macule — Circumscribed, non-elevated area of discoloration.

Pustule — Elevated area containing pus.

Sinus — a blind ended, usually epithelial lined, track. An attempt should be made to express pus from any sinus. The patency of a sinus should be tested using a probe or gutta percha cone.

Fistula — an epithelial lined tract running between two epithelial surfaces, e.g. mouth to maxillary antrum (oro-antral fistula).

- Record the site, shape, size and quality of the surface of any lesion.
- Draw the lesion and its site in the patient's notes. Record the lesion photographically, if possible.
- Palpate the lesion to determine whether it is soft, firm or hard, whether its edges are well defined or diffuse and whether the lesion is mobile or fixed.

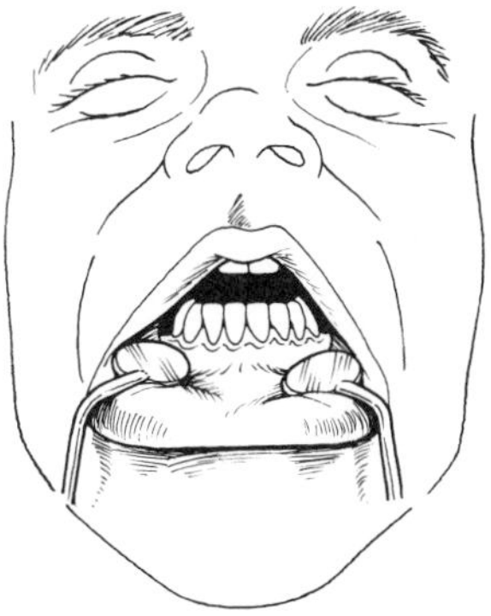

Figure 3.5 Retract the lips and examine the labial mucosa and sulcus with the mouth half open.

- Develop an order for examining the entire oral mucosa and use this routinely.

A suggested order for examination of oral mucosa is:

1. Upper and lower labial sulci. Retract the lips, with the mouth half open (Fig. 3.5).
2. Cheek mucosa. With the mouth wide open, retract the cheek (Fig. 3.6).
3. Upper and lower buccal sulci. Retract the cheek, with the mouth half open.

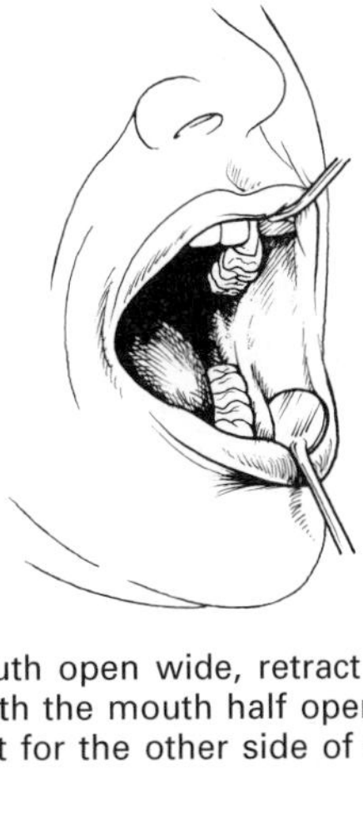

Figure 3.6 With the mouth open wide, retract the cheek and examine the buccal mucosa. Then with the mouth half open examine the maxillary and mandibular sulci. Repeat for the other side of the mouth.

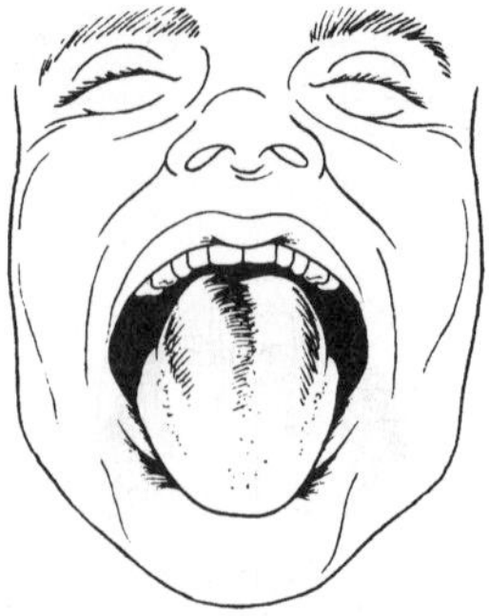

Figure 3.7 Inspect the tongue at rest and protruded.

4. Repeat 2 and 3 for the other side of the mouth.
5. Tongue. Dorsum — Inspect at rest and protruded (Fig. 3.7). Note any reduced mobility. Lateral border — Use gauze to hold the tip of the tongue and move it to one side (Fig. 3.8). Retract the cheek and view the lateral border of the tongue. Repeat for the other side.
6. Floor of the mouth and ventral surface of tongue (the commonest site for oral cancer). The floor should be viewed with the tip of the tongue raised to touch the palate (Fig.3.9).

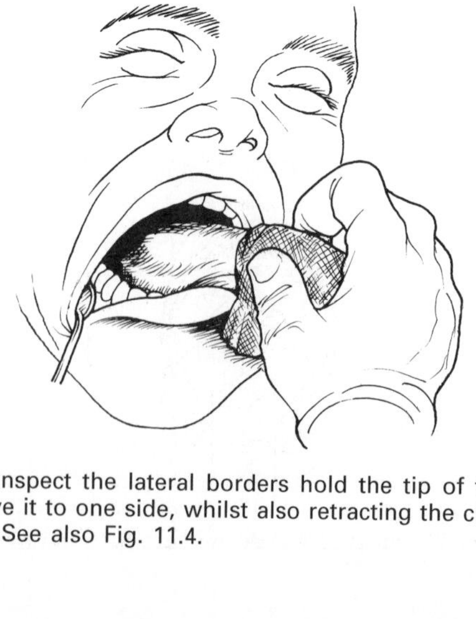

Figure 3.8 To inspect the lateral borders hold the tip of the tongue with gauze and move it to one side, whilst also retracting the cheek. Repeat for the other side. See also Fig. 11.4.

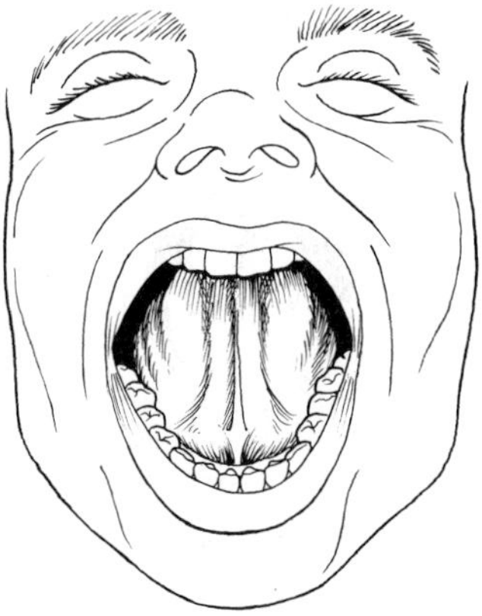

Figure 3.9 Examine the floor of the mouth and ventral surface of the tongue with the tip of the tongue touching the palate.

7. Palate (hard and soft). Depress the tongue using a tongue spatula (Fig. 3.10). Visually examine and palpate the hard palate. Visual examination of the soft palate includes its mobility. Request the patient to say 'Ah'.
8. Throat. Depress the tongue, again using a tongue spatula. Repeat the request to say 'Ah' and view the pillars of the fauces, tonsils, uvula and oropharynx.

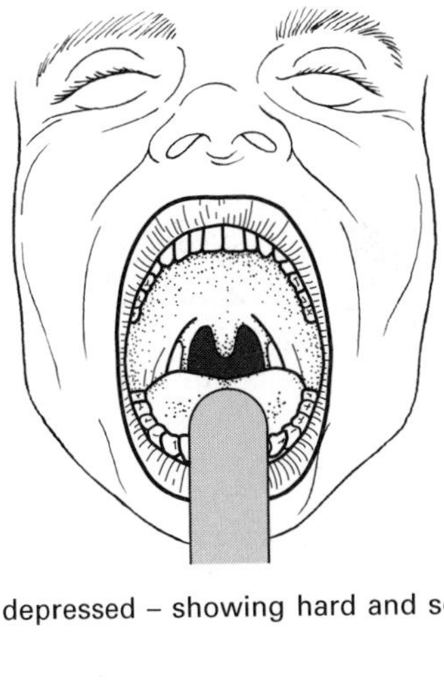

Figure 3.10 Tongue depressed – showing hard and soft palate.

Salivary glands

Use bimanual palpation of the submandibular glands and ducts to detect enlargement, tenderness or calculi (see Fig. 3.3).

Quality and consistency of saliva

Note the quantity of saliva expressed. Adhesion of the mirror to the buccal mucosa may indicate reduced salivary production. Bubbles of air in saliva are also suggestive of poor salivary production. Massage of normal major glands will produce a flow of saliva from the duct orifice. Note the quality and viscosity (e.g. sticky, tenaceous) of saliva, including any purulent discharge.

Periodontal examination

Note gingival colour and texture. Healthy gingivae are light pink, firm, knife-edged and stippled. Unhealthy gingivae are red, soft, swollen, glazed, smooth and may be ulcerated. Unhealthy gingivae will bleed following gentle probing or even spontaneously (see also Chapter 5). Use a periodontal pocket measuring probe to determine the distribution and severity of any pocketing.

Teeth

- Tooth mobility (Miller's classification).

Place the tips of the handles of two dental mouth mirrors onto the buccal and lingual surfaces of the tooth to measure mobility (Fig. 3.11).

Class 1 — Physiological mobility.
Class 2 — Up to 1 mm transverse movement.
Class 3 — More than 1 mm in any transverse direction or any non-physiological mobility on depression or rotation of the tooth.

Notes:

- Fremitus is the term given to non-physiological movement of a tooth during function.
- Teeth may be mobile as a result of periodontal disease, apical abscess, acute or chronic trauma, or other pathology of the soft or hard tissues.
- Dental charting.

The dental chart:
  Is a record of current status.

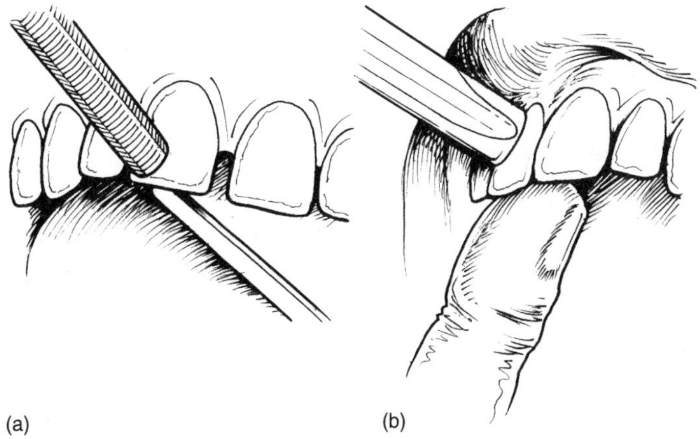

(a) (b)

Figure 3.11 Tooth mobility may be assessed using two instrument handles (a) or an instrument handle and a finger (b).

Aids treatment planning (if the chart accurately represents oral condition, e.g. size of lesion, priority etc.).
Facilitates third party communication.
Is a medicolegal requirement.
May be used for forensic purposes.

A routine must be established when examining the teeth, always starting in the same place and following the same sequence.

Absent teeth should be accounted for (i.e. extraction sites, unerupted teeth, teeth not developed).

Prior to examination, the teeth must be clean. This may entail scaling, flossing and polishing, if necessary. Saliva should be controlled by placement of cotton rolls in the sulci. Floss may also prove useful to detect overhangs, caries and open contacts between teeth.

- Diagnosis of dental caries:

Teeth must be cleaned, isolated and dried, as above. Good lighting is essential and can be augmented by transillumination (especially for suspected anterior approximal lesions), magnification and orthodontic tooth separators. The probe should be used mainly to remove debris and check for surface continuity. The probe must not be thrust into a suspected lesion or a cavity may be made where none existed. 'Stickiness' of a fissure to probing tells more about the sharpness and shape of the probe than the caries status of the fissure!

Look for cavitation, chalkiness, brown/blue/grey discoloration radiating peripherally under enamel from a pit or fissure or under a marginal ridge.

- Examination of existing restorations:

Look for approximal overhangs, marginal ditching, marginal gaps, fracture, wear, voids, contact relationship, marginal ridge height, recurrent caries and aesthetics. The chart should precisely reflect the size and shape of the restoration and the position and type of any problem identified.

- Examination for cracked cusps (see Chapter 5).
- Tooth surface loss (tooth wear) resulting from attrition, abrasion or erosion.
- Occlusion (static/functional). Includes examination for wear facets, fractured restorations or teeth, mobility, malpositioned, tilted teeth.

Static: Intercuspal position, Angle's classification:

Class I — Mesiobuccal cusp of maxillary first molar lies in the buccal groove of the mandibular first molar.

Class II — Mesiobuccal cusp of the maxillary first molar occludes mesial to the buccal groove of the mandibular first molar.
Division I — Anterior teeth proclined.
Division II — Anterior teeth retroclined.

Class III — Mesiobuccal cusp of the maxillary first molar occludes distal to the buccal groove of the mandibular first molar.

Also note coincidence/non-coincidence of centre lines, overbite (normally, the upper incisors should overlap the lower incisors by one-third of their clinical crown), overjet (normal range 2–3 mm), relationship of midlines, occlusal plane orientation, unopposed teeth, overerupted teeth, submerged teeth and plunger cusps.

Incisor relationship:

Class I — Lower incisor occludes with middle third of palatal surface of upper incisor.

Class II — Lower incisor occludes with cervical third of palatal surface of upper incisor.

Class III — Lower incisor occludes with incisal third of palatal surface of upper incisor.

Dynamic occlusion: Intercuspal position (ICP), retruded contact position (RCP) and the difference and direction between these, anterior guidance, canine guidance, group function, nonfunctional contacts e.g. non-working side interferences.

- Parafunction: Crenations (scalloped areas) on tongue/cheek. Tooth wear/tooth restoration fractures, masticatory muscle hypertrophy.

Edentulous ridge:
Note degree of resorption, any excess mobility of mucosa ('flabby ridge') and presence of any retained roots.

- Dentures: Kennedy classification, design, age, fit, retention, occlusion.

Having systematically considered the symptoms and signs, the available data may be passed through a diagnostic sieve such as the following:

The pathological (diagnostic/surgical) sieve:

Is the condition congenital or acquired?

Congenital:

Congenital lesions are often bilateral (e.g. torus mandibularis), acquired lesions are usually unilateral. (Lichen planus, however, typically presents bilaterally.)

Acquired:
Is the condition:

Infective?
Bacterial, fungal, viral, other
Acute or chronic

Neoplastic?
Benign, malignant
Primary, secondary

Traumatic?
Physical, chemical, electrical, thermal, electromagnetic

Metabolic?

Nutritional?

Drug-related?

Allergic?

Iatrogenic?

Psychological?

Degenerative?

Idiopathic?

Remember — common diseases occur commonly; exclude the most likely (e.g. pulpal pathology) before considering the rarity.

Conclusions

- Following the history and examination it is usually possible to form a provisional diagnosis.
- This will be confirmed or rejected by further diagnostic tests.

Notes:

- Never order tests that you cannot interpret. Always interpret tests that you have ordered.
- Any ulcer, lump, red or white patch that does not heal within 2 weeks requires immediate specialist referral.

Referral to a specialist (usually by letter):

- Supplementary verbal communication is usually very useful, e.g. with a local specialist or their registrar.

In an emergency, refer by telephone.

- **The referral letter should include:**

Name, address and telephone number of referrer.

Name, address, telephone number, age and gender of patient.

Date of referral.
Reason for referral, including case history, signs, symptoms and provisional diagnosis.
Suggested urgency of referral.
Medical, dental and social history.
Results of any special tests (including radiographs).
Request for opinion only or opinion and treatment.

Example referral letter:

Dr S Brown
The Dental Surgery
35 Dane End
London N1 3LP
Tel: 0208 773 2433

22nd February, 2000

Professor ......
Oral and Maxillofacial Surgery
The Guy's, King's and St Thomas' Dental Institute
Caldecot Road
London SE5 9RW

Dear Professor ......,

Re: Mr Charles White. D.O.B 17/2/20. 23 Elgin Court, London, N1 2JK. Tel: 0207 233 4455.

URGENT.

Mr White attended my surgery 10th February, 1998 for a routine check-up and did not complain of any dental problems. On examination of the left floor of the mouth I found a 5 mm diameter ulcer, with raised edges and a bleeding base. The ulcer was not particularly painful when touched but pressure on the lower denture in the area caused minor discomfort. I could detect no lymph node enlargement.

I relieved the lower denture and arranged to review the problem a week later.

At the review, the ulcer appeared unchanged. However, pressure on the lower denture still caused discomfort in the region of the ulcer. This time I cut the denture completely away from the ulcer site and arranged a second review.

At this second review, the ulcer shows no signs of healing and I am confident that the denture is not implicated. I am concerned that the ulcer may be malignant.

The medical history includes mild angina and chronic bronchitis only. Mr White takes no medication other than aspirin 75 mg and occasional use of glyceryl trinitrate.

Mr White has been edentulous for many years and wears complete upper and lower dentures. He smokes 20 cigarettes per day and drinks 4 or 5 glasses of whisky per week.

I should be grateful if you would examine Mr White urgently and provide any relevant treatment.

Yours sincerely,

Steven Brown

- Referrals can be made by facsimile. However, care should be taken to ensure a copy is also sent by post. Referrals should not be made by email, unless an encrypted system is being used.
- Patients should never be simply given a letter of referral and dispatched to the local specialist. This is discourteous to the specialist and to his/her other patients.

Further reading

Cooper, J., Warnakulasuriya, K.A.A.S. and Johnson, N.W. (1994) *Screening for Oral Cancer.* London: Royal College of Surgeons of England (Dept of Dental Sciences).

Gray, R.J.M., Davies, S.J. and Quayle, A.A. (1995) *Temporomandibular Disorders: A Clinical Approach.* London: British Dental Association.

4

Diagnostic tests

Summary

Introduction

Diagnostic tests

1. Routine 'dental' tests

- Vitality
  - Thermal
  - Electrical
  - Diagnostic access cavity
- Percussion
  - Tenderness
  - Percussion note
- Mobility
- Transillumination
- Magnification
- Photography
- Biting
- Auscultation
- Diagnostic local anaesthesia
- Temperature
- Radiography
- Simple techniques using radiopaque materials
  - Soft probes
  - Removable appliances

2. Routine 'medical' tests

- Temperature
- Blood pressure
- Pulse
- Respiratory rate
- Body weight

3. Additional tests

- Biopsy
- Biopsy methods
  - Excisional
  - Incisional
    - Scalpel
    - Punch
    - Needle/trephine/drill
    - Aspiration

continued

Microbiology (including virology)
Cytology
Blood
- Biochemistry
- Immunology

Cranial nerve tests

4. Referral

Advanced imaging techniques
- Computed tomography
- Magnetic resonance imaging
- Ultrasound

Advanced techniques using radiopaque materials:
- Arthrography
- Sialography
- Angiography
- Sinus/fistula investigation

Patch test
Urinalysis

Introduction

- Diagnostic tests should only be conducted after thorough history taking and examination (see Chapters 2 and 3).
- Tests are used to confirm or deny the provisional diagnosis in an attempt to arrive at a definitive diagnosis.
- Do not order a test if you will be unable to interpret the result!

Diagnostic tests

These tests are considered under the following four headings:

1. *Routine 'dental' tests.* These are part of the routine of the general dental practitioner.
2. *Routine 'medical' tests.* Simple medical examinations that may be conducted by a nurse or dentist trained in the techniques and able to interpret the results.
3. *Additional tests.* These may be undertaken in the dental surgery if the necessary equipment is available and personnel are suitably trained. If this is not the case, the patient should be referred to the appropriate centre. Again, the dentist must be able to interpret the results of any tests requested.

4. *Referral.* Tests which are not usually conducted in the general dental practice.

1. Routine 'dental' tests

Vitality tests (see also Chapter 5)

- These are used to attempt to determine the vitality (or non-vitality) of the dental pulp.
- When interpreted with the history and results of the examination, vitality tests may also provide a rough guide to states of inflammatory change of the pulp (pulpitis).
- However, results of pulp testing must be interpreted with caution; it only tests the integrity of the nerve supply in the pulp, while it is the blood supply that maintains pulpal health. Moreover, false positive and false negative results are common (see below).
- Vitality test results do not correlate well with histological changes occurring within the pulp.
- Testing should never be limited just to the tooth in question. Surrounding (supposedly healthy) and contralateral teeth should also be tested and the results compared.
- Testing should begin on a normal, healthy tooth, rather than a painful tooth or a tooth likely to provide an exaggerated response, to allay the patient's fears.
- Testing stimuli should be applied to normal enamel of the crown of the tooth, avoiding any restorations and soft tissues; while some restoratives are thermal conductors and may conduct to the soft tissues, others are thermal insulators.
- More reliable conclusions can be drawn if the results of two different tests are combined (e.g. heat and cold, or cold and electrical tests).

The following vitality tests are described:

Thermal
Electrical
Diagnostic access cavity, without anaesthesia

Thermal vitality tests

- A healthy tooth with a vital, non-inflamed pulp can usually be stimulated within a temperature range of some 20–50°C without pain.
- Teeth with inflamed pulps (pulpitis) may react with severe pain on temperature stimulation even within the above range.
- Extremes of temperature are employed in thermal vitality tests:

Cold A pledget of cotton-wool, held in college tweezers, is soaked in ethyl chloride. As the ethyl chloride evaporates, ice crystals form on the pledget. This process can be speeded up by application of an air-blast to the pledget, or waving the pledget in the air. The icy pledget is then applied to the tooth.

Heat A gutta-percha stick is heated in a flame until the tip softens. The hot tip is then applied to the tooth. If the tooth is previously lightly vaselined, the softened gutta-percha will not adhere to the tooth.

Electrical vitality tests These offer the advantage of a more controlled, graded stimulus in comparison with thermal tests, as most machines offer a digital display of the stimulus level. However, while this appears more accurate, variations occur, e.g. as the battery discharges.

The teeth to be tested must be isolated with cotton-wool rolls and dried. Any moisture on the tooth may conduct electricity into the soft tissues. The electrode in contact with a tooth should not be placed on a restoration; plastic restoratives are electrical insulators, while metals may conduct electricity to the gingival tissues or an adjacent tooth, for example. Likewise, the electrode must not contact soft tissues.

For reliable results, good electrical contacts must be made. An electrolyte (e.g. KY jelly) is usually required on the tip of the testing electrode and some machines require the operator to remove the latex glove from the hand holding the device, to provide a satisfactory earth.

The voltage should be gradually increased until a response is elicited.

Results of vitality testing These may be:

Positive (normal)
Exaggerated, brief
Exaggerated, prolonged
Negative
False positive
False negative
Inconclusive

Positive (normal):

- The test tooth responds in a similar way and to a similar level of stimulation to the other healthy teeth.
- This result suggests that the pulp is vital and not inflamed.

Exaggerated, brief:

- The test tooth responds more severely than other healthy teeth and/or to a lower level of stimulation.
- However, the painful response lasts for less than some 15 seconds after removal of the stimulus.
- The tooth may respond more to cold than heat stimulation.
- This result suggests that the pulp is vital but inflamed (hyperaemia, see page 80).
- The pulpitis may be reversible if the cause is eliminated.
- Alternatively, dentine may simply be exposed as a result of a crack, caries, leaking restoration or exposed and sensitive root dentine.

Exaggerated, prolonged:

- The test tooth responds more severely than other healthy teeth and/or to a lower level of stimulation.
- However, the painful response lasts for more than some 15 seconds (and occasionally minutes or even hours) after removal of the stimulus.
- The response to heat and electrical stimulation may be greater than to cold. Indeed, cold may reduce the pain.
- This result suggests that the pulp is vital but inflamed (acute pulpitis, see page 82). The pulpitis is likely to be irreversible.

Note: A very gradual reaction to heat, but not to cold or electrical stimulation, leading ultimately to an exaggerated response, may indicate chronic pulpitis (see page 83).

Negative:

- The test tooth does not respond to stimulation but healthy teeth do.
- This result suggests that the pulp is non-vital and may be necrotic, or that the root canals are sclerosed.

False positive:

- The test tooth responds normally but subsequent events prove the pulpal condition to be abnormal.
- This may occur:

In multi-rooted teeth; vital tissue remains in one root but the remaining pulp is necrotic.

In a root canal filled with pus; conducts stimuli (see apical periodontitis, page 85).

In a root canal filled with gas; heat causes expansion (see apical periodontitis, page 85).

A frightened patient, or a patient with a low pain threshold may report a painful response even before the stimulus is applied to the tooth!

False negative:

- The test tooth does not respond to stimulation but subsequent events prove the pulp to be vital.
- This may occur:

If the pulp is well insulated from thermal and electrical stimuli e.g. plastic restoration, secondary dentine. The latter partly explains the common occurrence of false negative responses from elderly teeth.

If the nerve supply to the pulp is damaged, e.g. trauma.

In patients with a high pain threshold.

With faulty technique or equipment.

Inconclusive:

- All teeth give exaggerated responses or, conversely, no teeth respond!
- Alternatively, different tests give conflicting results or the same test repeated subsequently gives conflicting results.
- If the results of two tests (e.g. heat and cold) are inconclusive, add a third test (e.g. electric). If doubt still exists, consider cutting a diagnostic access cavity, without local anaesthesia (see below).

Diagnostic access cavity without local anaesthesia

- Cutting a small cavity in the suspect tooth without anaesthesia is probably the most reliable vitality test.
- If the pulp is vital, a response is usually elicited as the dentine is entered.
- Since this test is destructive, it should be considered only as a last resort.

Percussion tests

- These are conducted by gently tapping a tooth with the tip of a dental mirror handle.
- Two characteristics are noted: tenderness to percussion, and a dull percussion note.
- Both characteristics denote inflammation of (and accumulation of fluid in) the periodontal ligament (see acute and chronic apical periodontitis, acute periodontitis of gingival origin and traumatic periodontitis, pages 85–88 and 90).

- Greater tenderness to percussion in an apical direction suggests apical periodontitis.
- Greater tenderness to percussion in a lateral direction suggests acute periodontitis of gingival origin (lateral periodontitis).
- Like vitality testing, a number of teeth should be tested in addition to the suspect tooth, and testing should begin on a healthy tooth.
- Percussion testing must be conducted with *great* care since teeth with periodontitis may be exquisitely tender.

Mobility

- Tooth mobility is assessed by use of two instrument handles one placed buccal and the other lingual on the tooth.
- Alternatively, a finger may substitute for one of the instruments (see page 27).
- Increased mobility is caused by:

Reduced bone support:
periodontal disease
bony cyst
neoplasm.

Abscess or inflammation of the periodontal ligament:
apical periodontitis
periodontitis of gingival origin
occlusal trauma
acute trauma.

Crown or root fracture.

Fracture of supporting bone.

Transillumination

- A dedicated light source may be purchased.
- Alternatively, a composite curing light can be employed.
- Less satisfactory is reflection of light from the operating lamp by a dental mirror.
- Transillumination is useful in the diagnosis of:

Tooth cracks.

Interproximal caries in anterior teeth.

Interproximal caries in posterior teeth, where there is sufficient access.

Intra-oral transillumination in a darkened room has been employed in the diagnosis of maxillary sinusitis.

Magnification
- Magnification (2×–4×) by lenses, loupes or video camera is generally useful to supplement naked eye examination of the oral cavity.
- It is particularly useful in the diagnosis of caries, tooth and restoration cracks, examination of restoration margins and identification of root canals during endodontic therapy.

Photography
- May magnify a lesion, facilitating diagnosis.
- Maintains a record of a lesion over time, enabling a more accurate judgement of healing or sinister change.
- May be helpful in medicolegal matters.

Biting
- Biting on a roll of rubber dam material, a rubber or wood point or dedicated, pyramidal shaped, plastic instrument may assist in the diagnosis of a cracked tooth (see page 78).

Auscultation
- A stethoscope placed over the temporomandibular joint may occasionally assist in the diagnosis of joint clicks or crepitus (see page 19).

Diagnostic local anaesthesia
- Dental pain, particularly that of pulpitis, is often very difficult to localize to the offending tooth (see page 81).
- Indeed, the patient may not even be certain from which jaw the pain arises.
- Elimination of pain, e.g. following a mandibular nerve block, or persistence of pain, localizes the cause to the correct jaw and may help to confirm a dental aetiology.
- Infiltration anaesthesia may be used to localize a causative tooth.

Temperature
- Should usually be measured using a clinical thermometer (see below).
- However, raised body temperature can be roughly gauged by placement of the back of the operator's ungloved hand on the patient's forehead.
- The temperature of an accessible facial swelling can be gauged by placing the backs of the operator's ungloved fingers on the swelling (Fig. 4.1).

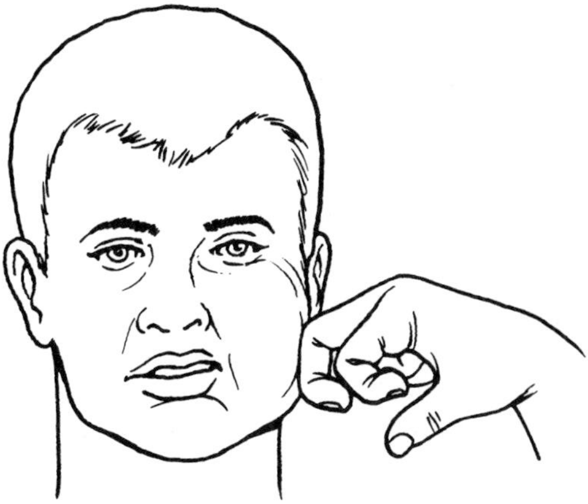

Figure 4.1 The temperature of an accessible facial swelling can be gauged by placing the backs of the operator's ungloved fingers on the swelling.

Radiography

- The following techniques are suitable for use in general dental practice where appropriate facilities exist:

Bitewing – Crowns of teeth, caries (particularly interproximal lesions), restorations, alveolar bone height (if bone loss is only modest). Extension of fissure caries into dentine will only be visible if the lesion is large.

Periapical – Root and surrounding bone.

***Parallax technique* (Fig. 4.2)**

- Two periapical films, exposed at slightly different anteroposterior angulation, assist in the assessment of the buccolingual position of unerupted teeth, particularly maxillary canines.
- The most *palatal* tooth appears to move in the *same* direction as the tube is moved.
- The most *buccal* tooth appears to move in the *opposite* direction to the tube.

Panoral – General view of teeth, jaws, temporomandibular joints, maxillary sinuses etc. Detail in the midline is obscured by superimposition of the cervical spine.

Lateral oblique – General view, as above. May be used where panoral facilities are not available.

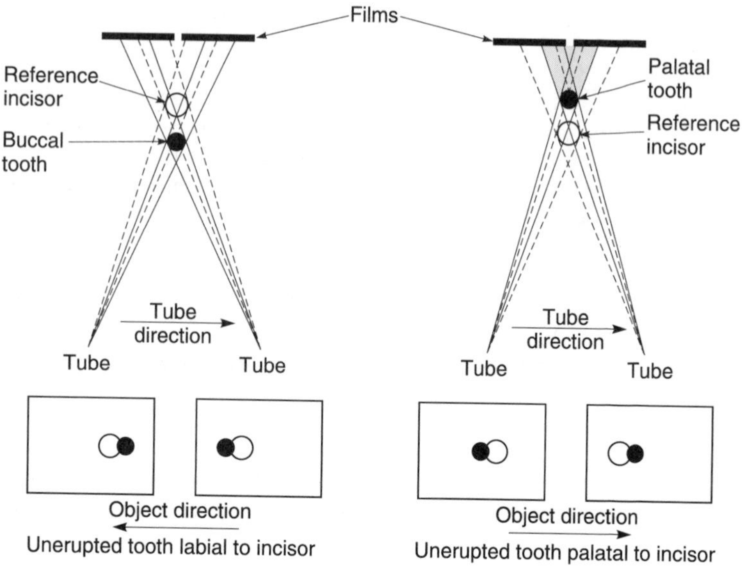

Figure 4.2 Localization by parallax: the more palatal object moves in the same direction as the tube; the more buccal object moves in a direction opposite to the tube.

Maxillary anterior occlusal – Roots of maxillary anterior teeth.

Mandibular occlusal – Calcification in the floor of the mouth, including submandibular gland and duct, buccolingual displacement of mandibular fractures.

Transpharyngeal – Temporomandibular joint.

Occipitomental – Maxillary sinuses, facial and skull bones.

Postero-anterior and lateral skull – Skull and facial bones. Useful in orthodontic assessment.

Stereoscopic radiography

- Two radiographs of the same area are taken but at a slightly different angle to each other.
- These are placed in a stereoscope and the mirrors adjusted until the two images come into focus, producing a 3D effect.
- The technique is particularly useful for detailed examination of fractures.

Simple techniques using radiopaque materials

Soft probes

- Soft probes (including endodontic silver or gutta-percha points) may be inserted along sinuses, e.g. dental sinuses to lead to the offending tooth apex and viewed radiographically.
- In a similar way, one or more needles may be inserted into tissue to localize a foreign body.

Removable appliances

- Wax base plates containing identifiable metal markers can be placed over the alveolus prior to recording a radiograph.
- This may be useful, e.g. in localizing a retained root at surgery.

2. Routine medical tests

The following tests may be undertaken in the dental surgery if the necessary equipment is available and personnel are suitably trained:

Temperature

- Body temperature, measured by sublingual placement (minimum 3 minutes) of a clinical thermometer, should be within the range 36.2–37.8°C. The thermometer must be shaken to reduce the mercury level to below 36°C prior to placement.
- Axillary temperature is slightly lower (and rectal temperature slightly higher) than sublingual temperature.
- Sublingual temperature should not be taken in infants since the glass may be chewed and broken.
- Body temperature varies slightly during the day, being higher during the evening than in the morning.
- Body temperature may be raised due to:
  Infection
  Surgery.
- Body temperature may be lowered due to:
  Hypothermia
  Severe shock.

Blood pressure

- Is measured using a sphygmomanometer.
- Is subject to wide variation within groups.
- Increases with increasing age.
- Is normally within the range 120–140 mmHg (systolic), 60–90 mmHg (diastolic).

- Raised diastolic pressure is more significant than raised systolic pressure.
- Raised blood pressure (hypertension, hyperpiesis) may be due to:
  Essential (idiopathic) hypertension (80%)
  Kidney disease (19%)
  Rare disorders (1%):
  Conn's disease
  Cushing's syndrome
  Phaeochromocytoma
  Coarctation of the aorta
  Raised intracranial pressure.
- A patient with raised blood pressure should be referred for full medical examination.
- Lowered blood pressure (hypotension) may be due to:
  Shock
  Haemorrhage
  Cerebrovascular accident
  Myocardial infarction.

Pulse

- Should be measured at both wrists since there may be variations between the sides.

Pulse rate

- In adults is normally 60–80 beats per minute.
- Is higher in infants (up to 140 beats per minute)
- May be lowered (bradycardia) in:
  Athletes
  Old age
  Hypothyroidism
  Heart block
  Vasovagal attack.
- May be raised (tachycardia) in:
  Thyrotoxicosis
  Infection
  Paroxysmal tachycardia
  Exercise
  Emotional upset.

Pulse rhythm

- The pulse should be regular.
- However, it tends to increase with inspiration and decrease with expiration.

- If this variation is marked, it is called 'sinus arrhythmia'.
- Common irregularities are extrasystoles which disappear on exercise. They are of no clinical significance.
- Atrial fibrillation is described as 'irregular irregularity' and is associated with serious problems including:
  Thyrotoxicosis
  Mitral stenosis
  Cardiac ischaemia.

Respiratory rate
- Normal adult respiratory rate is within 12–20 breaths per minute.
- Is faster in infants and slower in old age.
- Is increased by:
  Thyrotoxicosis
  Infections, particularly chest infections
  Pulmonary oedema
  Shock
  Exercise
  Emotional upset.
- May be decreased by:
  Rest and during sleep
  Narcotic drugs.

Cheyne–Stokes respiration
- Characterized by a repeating cycle of greatly reduced respiration (apnoea) followed by a gradually increasing rate to a maximum only to be followed by a gradual reduction to apnoea again.
- Cheyne–Stokes respiration is seen in the gravely ill:
  Cerebrovascular accident
  Meningitis
  Severe kidney disease.

Body weight
- A patient may be above or below the 'normal' weight.
- Sudden increase or loss of weight demands referral for full medical examination.
- Average body weight of populations in industrialized countries is increasing.
- Increase in body weight may be due to:
  Overeating
  Lack of exercise
  Pregnancy

Any condition causing fluid retention
Adverse reaction to drugs.

- Loss of weight may be due to:
  Anorexia nervosa
  Bulimia
  Diabetes mellitus
  Tuberculosis
  Thyrotoxicosis
  Malignancy
  Dieting.

3. Additional tests

The collection of specimens and conduct of some of the following tests may be undertaken in the dental surgery if the necessary equipment is available and personnel are suitably trained. If this is not the case, the patient should be referred to the appropriate centre. However, a referring practitioner still maintains a responsibility for the patient.

Biopsy

- Is the removal of tissue for further (usually histological) examination.
- Should be carried out whenever a suspicious lesion is encountered or a diagnosis cannot be made with any certainty.
- All intra-oral red lesions and non-removable white lesions should be biopsied (unless the diagnosis is certain and innocuous, e.g. aspirin burn).
- Any tissue that is excised should be sent for histological examination, even if the clinical dignosis seems reasonably certain.
- If the dentist is suspicious that a lesion may be malignant, the patient should be referred (urgently) for biopsy. In all other cases a specimen should be sent for examination.
- Biopsy specimens must be large enough for adequate histological examination; they should not be smaller than 1.0 cm × 0.5 cm.
- Avoid crushing, tearing and burning specimen (electrosurgery may make histological examination difficult).

Biopsy methods

Excisional
Incisional
  Scalpel
  Punch

Needle/trephine/drill
Aspiration

Excisional biopsy

- Usually applicable to discrete lesions, smaller than 1 cm diameter.
- Used only when the clinician is fairly certain that the lesion is benign.
- May risk shedding malignant cells if the provisional diagnosis of benign lesion is incorrect. However, the clinical value of biopsy far outweighs this risk.
- Constitutes the definitive treatment if the diagnosis of benign lesion proves correct.

Method: Administer local anaesthetic, by regional block where possible. In any event, local anaesthetic should not be closer than 2 cm from the site, to avoid 'waterlogging' of the specimen with anaesthetic solution.

Stabilize the lesion by transfixing it with a suture (Fig. 4.3). (Many specimens are ruined by crushing with tissue forceps.)

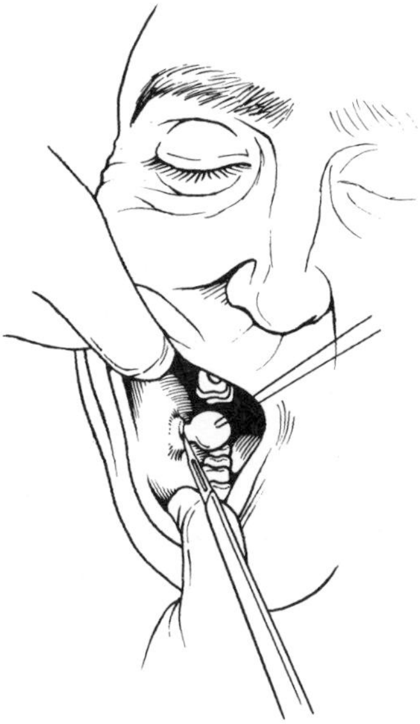

Figure 4.3 Excisional biopsy: stabilize the lesion by transfixing it with a suture. Stabilization by tissue forceps may damage the specimen.

Apply traction to the lesion via the suture.

Incise the mucosa around the base of the lesion in an elliptical shape.

Use a combination of blunt and sharp dissection to detach the lesion.

Place the specimen immediately in an appropriate, labelled, screw-top specimen bottle containing fixative (usually 10 times the specimen's volume of 10% formalin/formol saline).

Close the wound using sutures.

Incisional biopsy
- Applicable if the lesion is large or there is a suspicion of malignancy.
- May risk shedding malignant cells (see above).
- Incisional biopsy should *not* be performed on pigmented or vascular lesions. (Melanoma is highly metastatic and a vascular lesion may bleed excessively.)
- Record the position, size and shape of the lesion in the patient's record.

Method:
Administer local anaesthetic, as described above.

Identify the apparent junction between normal tissue and the lesion. Select the specimen across this region.

Stabilize the specimen with a suture (tissue forceps may crush the specimen).

Dissect the specimen from the edge of the lesion and include a margin of apparently normal tissue.

The specimen should include a representative area of the lesion.

Avoid necrotic areas of the lesion.

If the lesion is close to bone, avoid perforating the periosteum (this is to maintain the tissue boundary, in case the provisional diagnosis of benign lesion is incorrect).

Place the specimen immediately in a prescribed specimen bottle containing (usually) 10 times the specimen's volume of fixative (e.g. 10% formalin/formol saline).

Note: If specimens are to be subjected to immunofluorescent investigations, they should not be fixed. Instead they should be sent for immediate freezing at –70°C in liquid nitrogen.

Close the surgical site by sutures.

Punch biopsy

- A surgical instrument is used to punch out a representative portion of tissue.
- Since the resulting specimen is often damaged by the procedure, biopsy by scalpel is preferred.

Needle/trephine/drill biopsy

- These techniques have been employed to biopsy deep-seated fibro-osseous lesions.
- The resulting specimen is small, may be non-representative and again often damaged by the procedures; they are not often used.

Aspiration biopsy (see below for details of method)

- Is applicable to many cystic and fluctuant (i.e. fluid-containing) lesions.
- Failure to aspirate from a lesion suggests that it is solid.
- Is preferable to incisional biopsy of vascular lesions (e.g. haemangioma) due to the risk of excessive bleeding.
- Aspiration of air from the molar region of the maxilla suggests that the needle is in the maxillary sinus. This may help to differentiate the sinus from a possible cyst.
- Aspiration of air from a cystic mandibular lesion suggests a solitary (haemorrhagic) bone cyst (see page 175).
- Aspiration of blood suggests a haematoma, haemangioma or blood vessel.
- Aspiration of pus indicates an abscess or infected cyst.
- Aspiration of keratin, which looks like pus but has no unpleasant smell, indicates an odontogenic keratocyst (see page 166).
- Aspiration of a straw-coloured fluid containing crystals (of cholesterol) indicates a periodontal or dentigerous cyst (see pages 166, 168).
- The presence of keratin squames on microscopic examination of the aspirate from a cyst suggests odontogenic keratocyst (see page 166).

Microbiology

- Liaise with the testing laboratory to obtain swabs, specimen bottles, request forms etc., and details of preferred method of delivery and protective packaging.
- Specimens ideally should be taken before antimicrobial treatment is commenced.

- Allows the identification of organisms causing infections of dental origin.
- Organisms' sensitivity to various antibiotics can be determined, to facilitate the most effective treatment.

Note: Treatment of acute dental infections must be instituted before microbiological and antibiotic sensitivity test results are available.

- Where possible, samples of pus should be obtained by aspiration.

Method for aspiration biopsy:

Clean the tissue over the proposed aspiration site, using a mild antiseptic.

Inject local anaesthetic solution over (not into) the lesion.

Select a wide-bore needle and 10 ml syringe.

Penetrate the tissue and aspirate fluid.

Transfer the aspirate into a screw-top specimen bottle. (Do not fill the bottle more than two-thirds full.)

- If insufficient pus is available for aspiration, a swab should be used.

- Swab specimens should be taken at the time of surgical drainage.

Method for obtaining a swab specimen at the time of drainage:

Administer local anaesthetic if injection into inflamed tissues can be avoided. Otherwise use refrigeration anaesthesia by spraying ethyl chloride over the surface of the abscess. Alternatively, surface local anaesthesia or relative analgesia may be employed.

Make a drainage incision by cutting upwards with a No.11 blade (Fig. 4.4). (Cutting downwards with a No.15 blade will cause pressure in the abscess and pain, when refrigeration anaesthesia is used.)

Open the walls of the drainage incision for access for the swab by inserting the blades of sterile sinus forceps (Fig. 4.5).

An assistant should then insert the swab, take a sample of pus, then remove it without touching any other tissue.

Seal the swab in its container ensuring no contact of the swab with the external surface of the container or hand during insertion.

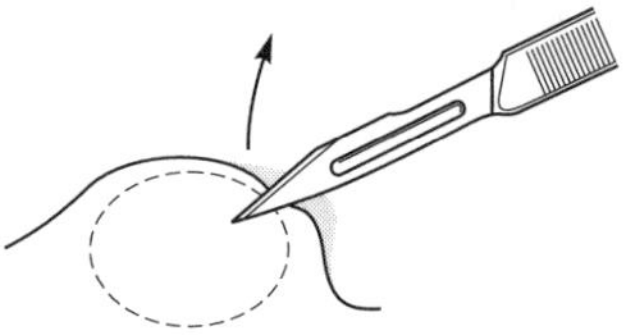

Figure 4.4 When using refrigeration anaesthesia (ethyl chloride spray) make the drainage incision by cutting upwards with a No. 11 blade.

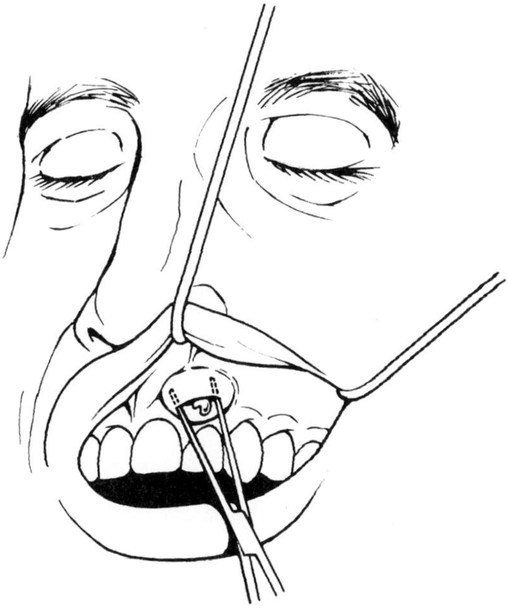

Figure 4.5 Method for obtaining a swab specimen at the time of surgical drainage: open the drainage incision for access for the swab by inserting sinus forceps blades.

Note: In suspected candidosis, the surface of the lesion or the related fitting surface of a denture may be swabbed.

Viral infections

- Swabs must be sent in a dedicated viral transport medium for culture or electron microscopy. Dry swabs are of no diagnostic value.

- A blood specimen (10 ml in a plain container) should also be taken for serology.
- Particular care must be taken with obtaining and transporting especially hazardous specimens, e.g. viral hepatitis, HIV. Contamination of the external surfaces of the specimen tube and needlestick injury must obviously be avoided.

Exfoliative cytology

- Is the microscopic study of cells exfoliated or scraped from the surface of a lesion.
- Is an adjunct to biopsy, not a substitute.
- Is indicated when biopsy cannot be undertaken, is refused by the patient, where multiple lesions need investigation, or where serial specimens need to be taken frequently over long periods.
- If interpretation of a cytological specimen is in doubt, a biopsy is indicated.

Method: Do not wipe the surface of the lesion except to remove necrotic material.

Ensure the surface of the lesion is moist. (Do not dry the surface.)

Scrape the surface of the lesion with the edge of a sterile flat plastic instrument or moistened wooden tongue spatula.

The scraping action should be repeated several times in the same direction.

The scrapings obtained should be transferred to a previously labelled microscope slide and spread over the slide surface using the edge of another slide.

Immediately fix the specimen using an appropriate fixative (e.g. 10% formalin/formol saline).

Labelling of specimen bottles and completion of request forms:

- All specimen bottles must be labelled with the patient's details.
- Specimens must be accompanied by a completed request form.
- The request form should include details of the provisional diagnosis, history of any antimicrobial therapy and any drug allergies.
- The request form must also include adequate clinical information to allow accurate interpretation of the test results.
- These may include: a diagram of the specimen; clinical features (size, site, colour, consistency, mobility, associated lymphadenopathy, etc.).

Notes

1. In suspected syphilis (see pages 148, 189, 219), oral lesions should be cleaned with saline before a smear is made for dark ground examination. A blood specimen (10 ml in a plain container) should also be sent for RPR and TPHA testing.
2. If tuberculosis is suspected this must be stated on the request form.

Transportation of clinical/pathological specimens:

A triple packaging system should be used (primary container, secondary container, outer packaging):

- Specimens must be collected into the appropriate primary container.
- The primary container must be leak proof.
- Liquid specimens must not fill the primary container at 55°C.
- The primary container must be labelled appropriately.
- The primary container must be placed into a watertight secondary container.
- For liquid specimens, sufficient absorbent material to absorb the entire contents of the primary container must be placed between the primary and secondary container.
- The primary and secondary containers must be placed into an outer package.
- The request form must be properly filled in.
- Between the secondary container and the outer package, the following details are required:
  An itemized list of contents
  The request form
  Name and address of the recipient
  Name and address of the sender
  Contact telephone number.
- On the outer packaging include:
  Name and address of the recipient
  Name and address of the sender
  A contact name with an emergency contact number
  An 'Infectious Substance' sticker.
- When possible, specimens should be delivered to the laboratory by hand. Specimens transported through the post may be damaged, delayed or lost.
- Specimens sent with the Royal Mail must be placed in United Nation Class 6.2 specification packaging and comply with U.N.602 packaging requirements (packaging and details obtainable from the Royal Mail).

Blood

Venepuncture

- Liaise with the haematological laboratory to obtain report sheets, blood specimen bottles and information relating to the quantity of blood required for the tests.
- Blood for film, red cell indices, white cell and platelet counts is usually collected in an EDTA tube. (The EDTA prevents the specimen clotting.)
- Blood for Paul–Bunnell test (see page 152), serum iron and blood grouping is usually collected in a plain tube.
- Blood for ESR and prothrombin time is usually collected in a citrated tube.

Method

- The site for venepuncture is usually at the level of the elbow of the arm, the antecubital fossa.
- The preferred site is the lateral aspect of the antecubital fossa.
- The medial aspect of the antecubital fossa may also show prominent veins but a superficial branch of the brachial artery may also be present and is to be avoided.
- The basilic and cephalic veins (Fig. 4.6) are joined by the median cubital vein. If the median cubital vein is V-shaped, the two arms of the V are the median basilic and median cephalic veins.
- The median basilic vein is the usual site for venepuncture. However, select a vein that can be felt as well as seen.
- Palpate the vein to confirm that it is indeed a vein and not an artery. Arteries will be felt to pulsate, veins will not.
- Support the patient's arm on a table or the arm of the dental chair and extend the elbow.
- Apply a tourniquet or sphygmomanometer cuff (inflated to 80 mmHg) to the upper arm.

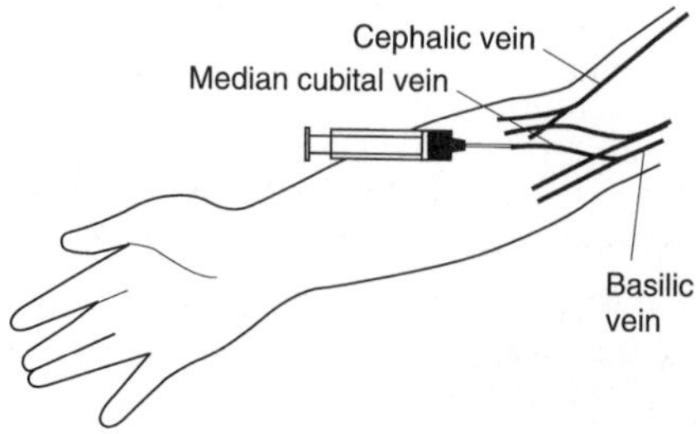

Figure 4.6 The site for venepuncture is usually the antecubital fossa.

- Distend the veins by asking the patient to clench the fist several times. Further distension can be achieved by lightly tapping the skin over the veins.
- Clean the proposed puncture site with an antiseptic swab.
- Steady the vein by stretching the skin over the vein with the fingers of one hand.
- Puncture the skin 1 cm distal to the site at which the lumen is to be entered.
- The needle should be bevel uppermost, should lie parallel to the vein, and be held at an angle of 30 degrees to the skin.
- The fact that the lumen has been entered is confirmed by withdrawal of blood when the plunger of the syringe is withdrawn.
- Aspirate the required quantity of blood.
- Hold an antiseptic swab over the puncture site and withdraw the needle.
- Exert pressure over the site when the needle has been withdrawn, to prevent haematoma formation. The patient can maintain this pressure for a few minutes simply by flexing the forearm.

A full blood count measures:

Red cell count
Haemoglobin
Packed cell volume (haematocrit)
Mean cell volume
Mean cell haemoglobin
Mean cell haemoglobin concentration
White cell count
Platelet count

Data Red cell count (RBC): Males 4.2–6.1 $\times$ 10^{12}/l, females 4.2–5.4 $\times$ 10^{12}/l. Raised in polycythaemia, lowered in anaemia.

Haemoglobin (Hb): Males 13.5–18 g/dl, females 11.5–16.5 g/dl. Raised in polycythaemia, lowered in anaemia and after haemorrhage.

Packed cell volume (PCV) (Haematocrit, Hct): Males 40–54%, females 37–47%. Raised in polycythaemia, lowered in anaemia.

Mean cell volume (MCV): 79–96 fl. Raised (macrocytosis) in B_{12} and folate deficiency and alcoholism, lowered (microcytosis) in iron deficiency anaemia.

Mean cell haemoglobin (MCH): 27–31 pg. Determined by dividing haemoglobin (Hb) by the red cell count (RBC). Raised in pernicious anaemia, lowered in iron deficiency anaemia.

Mean cell haemoglobin concentration (MCHC): 32–36 g/dl. Determined by dividing haemoglobin (Hb) by the packed cell volume (PCV). Lowered in iron deficiency anaemia (for which it is the most reliable test).

White cell count (WBC/WCC): 4–11 × 10^9/l. Raised in leukaemia and infection, lowered (leucopenia) in immunosuppression, aleukaemic leukaemia, aplastic anaemia and some viral infections.

Neutrophils: approx. 3 × 10^9/l. Raised with infection, trauma and malignancy. Lowered by some drugs and bone marrow disease.

Lymphocytes: approx. 2.5 × 10^9/l. Raised in leukaemia and glandular fever. Lowered by immune defects (e.g. HIV, AIDS).

Monocytes: approx. 0.6 × 10^9/l. Raised in monocytic leukaemia and glandular fever. Lowered by immune defects.

Eosinophils: approx. 0.15 × 10^9/l. Raised with allergy and all parasitic diseases. Lowered by immune defects.

Platelets (PLT): 150–400 × 10^9/l. Raised (thrombocytosis) in chronic inflammatory conditions and myeloproliferative disease, lowered (thrombocytopenia) in HIV, leukaemia and connective tissue diseases.

Erythrocyte sedimentation rate (ESR): 0–15 mm per hour. A raised ESR is an important non-specific indicator of disease, ranging from infection to malignancy.

Reticulocytes: Constitute up to 6% of RBC (children), up to 1.5% RBC (adults). Raised with increased marrow activity (e.g. after haemorrhage).

Coagulation screening

Prothrombin International Normalized Ratio (INR): Normal range 0.9–1.2.

Prothrombin Time (PT): Normally less than 1.3.

Activated Partial Thromboplastin Time (APTT) ratio: Normal range 0.85–1.15.

Fibrinogen level: Normal range 1.5–4.5 g/l.

Factor VIII level: Normal range 50–150 u/dl.

(Haematology report may mark abnormal results low (L), high (H) or critical (C)).

Blood film terminology

- A normal red cell is described as normocytic (normal size) and normochromic (normal colour).

Abnormalities of size and shape include:

Macrocyte – Red cell larger than normal (e.g. vitamin B_{12}, folate deficiency).

Megaloblast – Nucleated red cell larger than normal (e.g. megaloblastic anaemia).

Microcyte – Red cell smaller than normal (e.g. iron deficiency).

Anisocytosis – Red cells vary in size (e.g. iron deficiency).

Poikilocytosis – Red cells vary in shape (e.g. iron deficiency).

Sickle cell – Sickle-shaped red cell (e.g. sickle-cell anaemia).

Acanthocyte – Red cell with a spiky projection (e.g. haemolytic anaemia).

Spherocyte – Red cell spherical in shape (e.g. hereditary spherocytosis).

Abnormalities of colour:

Hypochromia – Pale red cells (reduced haemoglobin content) (e.g. iron deficiency).

Anisochromia – Irregular staining (e.g. severe anaemia).

Polychromasia – Red cells vary in staining (e.g. following blood loss).

Target cell – Pale red cell with aggregation of haemoglobin in the centre (like an archery target) (e.g. iron deficiency).

Abnormality of shape and colour:

Leptocyte – Red cell thin and pale (e.g. thalassaemia).

Immature red cells:

Blasts – Nucleated precursors are not normally present (except in the newborn infant). Their presence suggests severe anaemia, leukaemia, multiple myeloma.

Myelocytes

Metamyelocytes (e.g. malignant bone marrow disease)

Promyelocytes

Normoblasts

Reticulocytes (e.g. haemolysis).

Blood biochemistry

- Contact the laboratory to determine the quantity of blood required and the appropriate specimen tube.
- Most biochemical tests can be carried out on serum. Thus, blood should be collected in a plain tube.
- For analysis of electrolytes and proteins, plasma is required and blood should be collected in a lithium heparin tube.
- For blood glucose analysis, blood should be collected in a fluoride bottle.

Data Acid phosphatase (0–13 IU/l). Raised in acute myeloid leukaemia and pancreatic cancer.

Alkaline phosphatase (30–110 IU/l). Raised in Paget's disease, fibrous dysplasia, hyperparathyroidism and bone malignancy. Lowered in hypothyroidism.

Calcium (2.3–2.6 mmol/l). Raised in hyperparathyroidism, bone malignancy and sarcoidosis. Lowered in hypoparathyroidism and rickets.

Phosphate (0.8–1.7 mmol/l). Raised in bone disease, lowered in hyperparathyroidism.

Ferritin (serum iron) (25–190 ng/ml male, 15–99 ng/ml female). Raised in leukaemia, lymphoma and other malignancies. Lowered in iron deficiency anaemia.

Folic acid (3–20 μg/l). Lowered in dietary deficiency, alcoholism, haemolytic anaemia and certain drugs, e.g. phenytoin.

Glucose (2.8–5.0 mmol/l). Raised in diabetes mellitus.

Vitamin B_{12} (150–800 ng/l). Raised in leukaemia, lowered in pernicious anaemia, dietary deficiency.

Blood immunology

- Most tests are carried out on serum and blood should usually be collected in a plain tube.
- However, serum for some tests requires special handling. Details should be obtained from the laboratory.
- Autoantibodies of interest to the dentist include:

Epithelial basement membrane – Pemphigoid

Epithelial intercellular cement – Pemphigus

Rheumatoid factor – Rheumatoid arthritis
– Systemic lupus erythematosus

Salivary duct antibody – Sjögren's syndrome

- Immunoglobulins:

IgG – raised in pemphigus, myelomatosis and connective tissue diseases.

IgG, IgA and IgM – all lowered in immunodeficiency states.

Cranial nerve tests

I. Olfactory nerve

Responsible for the perception of smell.

- Loss of smell (anosmia) is more often due to nasal mucosal inflammation than olfactory nerve damage.
- Thus, the patient should first be questioned about nasal discharge.
- The patency of the nasal passages may be tested by asking the patient to sniff, as each nostril is closed in turn by finger pressure.
- However, olfactory nerve damage may occur with fractures of the ethmoid bones or a tumour of the anterior cerebral fossa.

Test:

The patient (with eyes closed or blindfold) is asked to identify various common substances by smell only. Substances may include lemon, peppermint etc.

Each nostril is tested separately, the other being occluded.

- Altered perception of smell may also occur with:

Phenytoin
Epilepsy
Migraine
Depression (and other psychological/psychiatric conditions).

II. Optic nerve

Responsible for vision.

Visual acuity:

- Visual acuity is assessed (usually following referral) using Snellen's charts placed at 6 m from the patient.

Visual fields:

- Visual fields are assessed by the 'confrontation' test, where the patient's field of vision is compared to that of the clinician (Fig. 4.7).

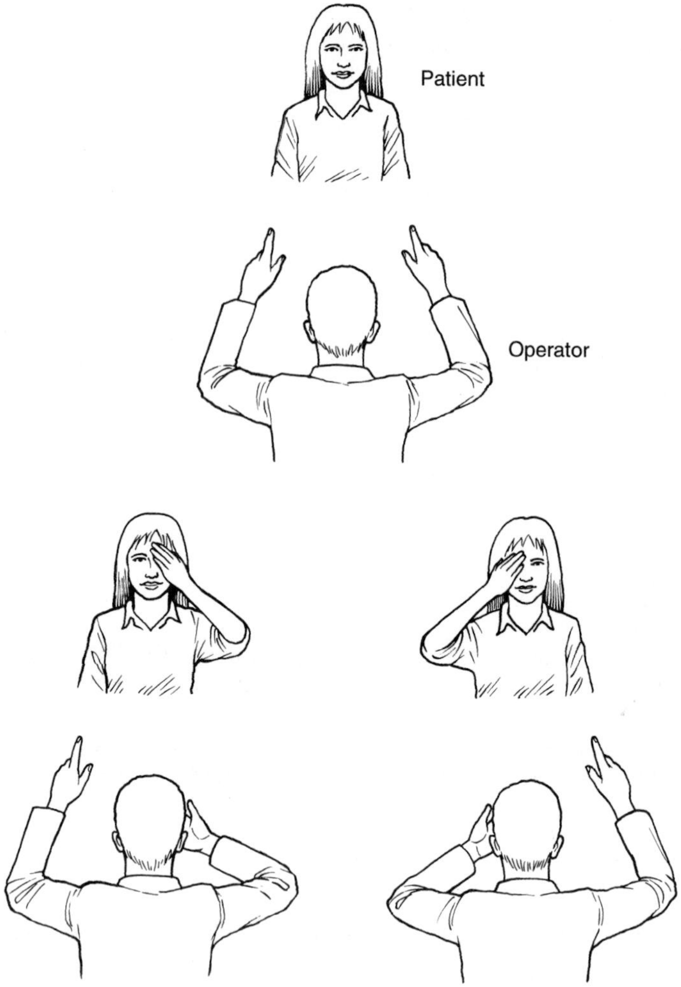

Figure 4.7 Testing the visual fields: 'confrontation' test.

Method

The clinician sits opposite the patient, approximately 1 m away, with eyes at the same level.

The patient covers the left eye and stares with the right eye into the clinician's left eye. At the same time, the clinician covers his right eye and stares into the patient's right eye.

The clinician then places his left hand with a finger outstretched outside the periphery of his field of vision and between himself and the patient.

The finger is then drawn into the clinician's field of vision and the patient asked to report when the clinician's finger becomes visible.

Each eye is tested in this way to include the nasal, temporal, superior and inferior fields.

Light reflex:

- The light reflex is tested by shining a light into the patient's eye.
- The pupil of the eye into which the light is shone should constrict (direct reflex), as should the pupil of the other eye, in which no light is shone (consensual reflex).
- Failure of a pupil to constrict may be due to:

Failure to detect light (optic nerve damage)
Autonomic dysfunction
Drugs
Head injury
Coma
Death!

- Pupils are normally round, regular in shape and equal in size.
- Pupil size varies with ambient light but is usually within 3–5 mm.
- Constriction of the pupil below 3 mm is termed miosis.
- Dilatation above 5 mm is termed mydriasis.

III. Oculomotor nerve

Is the motor supply to all the extra-ocular muscles except superior oblique and lateral rectus.

The oculomotor nerve also contains motor fibres to levator palpebrae superioris (which elevates the upper eyelid) and parasympathetic fibres to sphincter pupillae (to constrict the pupil).

- Thus, oculomotor nerve damage leads to :

Drooping of the upper eyelid (ptosis)
Poor up, down and inward eye movement leading to –
Double vision (diplopia)
Dilated pupil, non-reactive to light.

Test for eye movements

The patient should face the clinician and be asked to follow the movements of the clinician's finger held approximately half a metre away, with the patient's head still.

The clinician's hand should be moved medially and laterally, upwards and laterally, upwards and medially, downwards and medially, and downwards and laterally.

IV. Trochlear nerve

Provides motor supply to superior oblique extra-ocular muscle.

The superior oblique muscle is a pure depressor of the eye when the eye is adducted (turned inwards).

- Thus, damage to the trochlear nerve causes:

Inability to look downwards and inwards
Diplopia

V. Trigeminal nerve

The trigeminal nerve has three main divisions:

Ophthalmic
Maxillary
Mandibular

Each division contains sensory fibres to supply the orofacial tissues, including oral, nasal, conjunctival and sinus mucosa and part of the tympanic membrane.

The mandibular division also contains motor fibres to the muscles of mastication.

Testing of sensory function

Hold a pledget of cotton wool in college tweezers and tease out a few wisps to form a point.

With the patient's eyes closed, lightly touch the area of tissue under investigation with the cotton wool point and ask the patient if any sensation is felt.

Repeat the test on equivalent tissue on the other side of the face.

If any loss of sensation is detected, map out the area affected.

Then confirm the results by repeating the test (gently) with a sharp point such as the tip of a dental probe.

Testing of motor function

Ask the patient to fully open and close the mouth, move the jaw to the left and right, then forward and back. (Normal limits of mandibular movement are detailed on page 18).

Weakness in movement can be assessed by the clinician providing resistance to movement by placing a hand on the patient's jaw.

- Two reflexes should be demonstrated when testing the trigeminal nerve:

i) Corneal reflex
ii) Jaw jerk

Corneal reflex:

Ask the patient to look to the side.

Lightly touch the cornea with a wisp of cotton wool, without the patient being able to see the approach of the cotton wool.

In health, the eye lids of both eyes should blink.

Repeat for the other eye.

Jaw jerk reflex (Fig. 4.8):

The patient is asked to open the lips and relax the jaw.

Place a thumb on the patient's chin, just below the lower lip.

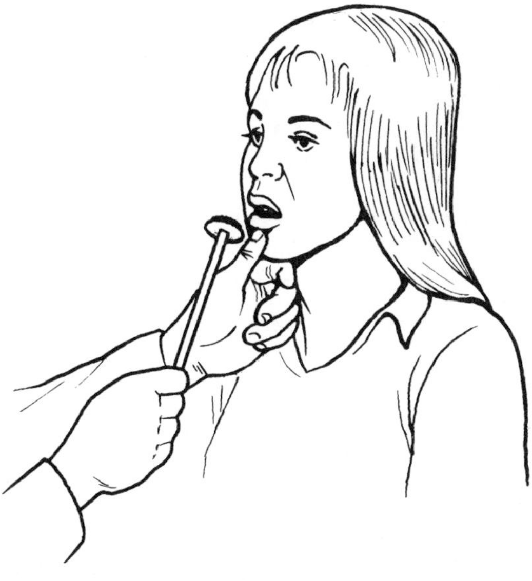

Figure 4.8 Eliciting the jaw jerk reflex.

Sharply tap the thumb with a tendon hammer (if available) or the fingers of the other hand.

The patient's jaw should close.

VI. Abducens nerve
Supplies motor fibres to the lateral rectus extra-ocular muscle.

The lateral rectus muscle moves the eye laterally.

- Thus, damage to the abducens nerve causes paralysis of lateral eye movement (abduction).

Test
See test for eye movement (above).

VII. Facial nerve
Supplies:

Motor fibres to the muscles of facial expression.
Motor fibres to the stapedius muscle in the middle ear.
Sensory taste fibres from the anterior two-thirds of the tongue.
Secretomotor fibres to the submandibular, sublingual and lacrimal glands.

- The lower facial muscles are unilaterally innervated, while the upper muscles are bilaterally innervated.
- Signs of facial paralysis are often obvious on inspection and include:

Absence of wrinkles on the forehead
Drooping of the corner of the mouth
Flattening of the nasolabial fold

Testing of facial nerve motor function
Ask the patient to smile, frown, whistle, blow out the cheeks, close the eyes tightly and 'screw up' the face.

Next, ask the patient to raise each eyebrow in turn.

- Damage to the facial nerve will lead to inability to perform the above on one side of the face.
- If the patient exhibits unilateral facial muscle paralysis, but is able to raise both eyebrows, damage is likely to be an upper motor neurone lesion (see page 106).

Upper motor neurone lesions:

Cerebrovascular accident

Neoplasm
Demyelinating disease

- If the eyebrow on the affected side cannot be raised, damage is likely to be a lower motor neurone lesion.

  Lower motor neurone lesion:

Bell's palsy (see page 105).

Test for taste perception
Prepare dilute solutions representing the four primary tastes (sweet, salt, sour, bitter). These may include solutions of:

Sugar
Table salt
Vinegar
Quinine

Ask the patient to protrude the tongue and hold the tip of the tongue forward, using a gauze swab.

Apply the test solution to the lateral borders of the anterior two-thirds of the tongue. Ask the patient to identify the taste (i.e. 'sweet', 'salt', etc.).

Allow the patient to rinse with water, then repeat with the next test solution.

VIII. Vestibulocochlear nerve
Is made up of two parts:

Cochlear component – Sensory for hearing
Vestibular component – Sensory for balance

Definitive testing of the vestibulocochlear nerve is beyond the remit of the dentist.

However, a crude assessment of hearing may be made by asking the patient to repeat words whispered into the ear, while the other ear is covered.

A crude assessment of balance may be made by asking the patient to stand on one leg or walk along a fine line.

IX. Glossopharyngeal nerve
Supplies:

Sensory fibres to the posterior third of the tongue (including taste), pharynx, middle ear and eustachian tube.

Motor fibres to the stylopharyngeus muscle.
Secretomotor (parasympathetic) fibres to the parotid gland.

Test
Testing of the glossopharyngeal nerve is based on the gag reflex, which also involves the vagus nerve (efferent path).

Gag reflex:
Ask the patient to open the mouth widely.

Touch the pharyngeal tissue lightly with the tip of a wooden spatula.

In health, this should result in bilateral elevation of the soft palate.

Needless to say, this is an unpleasant procedure and should only be conducted when glossopharyngeal nerve damage is suspected.

X. Vagus nerve
Supplies:

Motor fibres to the muscles of the palate, larynx and pharynx.
Sensory fibres from the viscera of the thorax and abdomen.
Autonomic fibres to the bronchi, heart and gastrointestinal tract.

Testing of the oropharyngeal component of the vagus nerve:
Ask the patient to open the mouth widely and say a prolonged 'Ah'.

In health, this should result in equal bilateral elevation of the soft palate.

If the nerve is unilaterally damaged, the soft palate deviates to the healthy side and elevation is unequal.

If the voice is hoarse, the patient should be referred for laryngoscopy.

XI. Spinal accessory nerve
Supplies:

Motor fibres to the sternomastoid and trapezius muscles.

Test for sternomastoid function
First, ask the patient to press the chin downwards while the clinician provides resistance by placing a hand beneath the patient's chin.

The definition and apparent size of the two sternomastoid muscles should be approximately equal.

Then ask the patient to turn the head to one side while the clinician provides resistance against the movement by placing a hand against the patient's jaw.

In health, the contralateral sternomastoid muscle should contract and be clearly visible beneath the skin.

Repeat for the other side.

Test for trapezius function
Ask the patient to shrug the shoulders while the clinician provides resistance against the movement by placing a hand on each shoulder.

XII. Hypoglossal nerve
Supplies:

Motor fibres to the extrinsic and intrinsic muscles of the tongue, except palatoglossus.

Test
Ask the patient to protrude the tongue.

In health, the tongue should protrude in the midline.

If the hypoglossal nerve is damaged unilaterally, the tongue will deviate to the damaged side.

Muscular power of the tongue can be assessed by asking the patient to push the tip of the tongue into the cheek while the clinician provides resistance by placing a finger on the overlying cheek.

4. Referral

The conduct of the following tests is not usually undertaken in the dental surgery; instead, the patient is referred to the appropriate centre.

As detailed above, the referring practitioner still maintains a responsibility for the patient and must be able to interpret the results of any tests requested.

Advanced imaging techniques

Computed tomography (CT)
- Increasingly allows three-dimensional image reconstructions.
- Allows exact visualization of the shape and size of a lesion and proximity to important structures.

- May be used to image the major salivary glands.
- Is very useful in the planning of surgery, particularly prior to implant placement.
- However, CT scans require a high radiation dose.

Magnetic resonance imaging (MRI)

- May be used to image the major salivary glands.
- Less satisfactory than computed tomography for imaging bones.

Ultrasound

- Particularly useful for examination of cysts and space-occupying lesions.
- Can also be used to visualize the temporomandibular joints and major salivary glands.

Advanced techniques using radiopaque materials

Arthrography:

- Injection of contrast media into the upper and lower compartments of the temporomandibular joint.
- May be combined with cineradiography to observe joint movements.

Sialography

- Injection of contrast medium into the ducts of the major salivary glands.
- May be followed by conventional radiography or computed tomography.
- Will demonstrate:

Glandular structure, e.g. glandular dilatation (sialectasis)
Intra-glandular lesions
Duct obstruction, e.g. calculi
Duct restriction (stricture)
Duct dilatation

- Prior to sialography, the medical history must include questioning about allergy to iodine; some contrast media contain iodine.

Angiography

- Injection of radiopaque material into the blood stream.
- Useful for demonstrating aneurysms and arteriovenous shunts.
- The latter may rarely cause radiolucent areas in the jaws.

Sinus/fistula investigation

- Contrast media can be injected into sinuses and fistulae to determine their path and extent.

Patch test

- Skin patch tests may be employed to test for allergy to substances that may be used in dentistry.
- Increasingly, patients are concerned with possible allergy to dental amalgam.
- True allergy to dental mercury and other components of amalgam (and other dental materials) is rare but does occur.
- Patch testing and interpretation of the results should be undertaken by a competent dermatologist.
- Test kits designed for use in the dental surgery, with the results interpreted by the dentist (or other untrained personnel), are unreliable.

Urinalysis

- Normal daily urine output in a healthy adult is approximately 1500 ml.
- Water excretion is usually impaired after surgery or severe accident, and increased in diabetes insipidus and with use of diuretics.
- The following substances are not usually found in the urine of the healthy subject; their presence may indicate disease:

Proteins (proteinuria):

- May be due to:
  Infection of the urinary tract (cystitis, pyelitis)
  Most kidney diseases
  Multiple myeloma (Bence–Jones protein)

Note: A trace of protein is a frequent contaminant of urine samples.

Cells:

- If urine is examined microscopically, occasional cells will often be seen.
- However, urine should not contain more than 1 red cell and 15 white cells per cubic millimetre.

Blood (haematuria):

- May be caused by trauma or disease of the kidney or from the renal tract.
- Should be tested for in all accident cases.

Glucose (glycosuria):

- May be found in diabetes mellitus (acetone also present)

Pus (pyuria):

- May be found in any infection of the urinary tract.

Bilirubin:

- May be found with jaundice.

Further Reading

Scully, C. and Cawson, R.A. (1998) *Medical problems in dentistry*. 4th edn. Oxford: Wright.

Pain of dental origin

Summary

Differential diagnosis

1. Pulpal pain

Exposure of dentine, such as:
Root dentine hypersensitivity
Caries
Defective restoration
Fractured or cracked tooth

Pulpitis
Initial pulpitis (hyperaemia)
Acute pulpitis
Suppurative pulpitis (pulpal abscess)
Chronic pulpitis
Chronic hyperplastic pulpitis (pulp polyp)

Galvanism
Aerodontalgia
(See also Atypical odontalgia, Chapter 6)

2. Periodontal pain

Acute apical periodontitis of pulpal origin
Traumatic periodontitis
Chronic apical periodontitis of pulpal origin
Acute periodontitis of gingival origin (periodontal/parodontal abscess)
Periodontal-endodontic lesion

3. Gingival pain

Traumatic gingivitis
Acute necrotising ulcerative gingivitis (ANUG)
Herpetic gingivostomatitis (see Chapter 8)
Pericoronitis (including 'teething')
'Desquamative' gingivitis:
Lichen planus (see Chapters 10 and 11)
Mucous membrane pemphigoid (see Chapter 10)

4. Bone pain

Dry socket (osteitis)
Osteomyelitis (see Chapter 8)
Infected dental cyst (see Chapter 9)
Trauma, fracture (see Chapter 7)

5. Pain associated with denture bases

Introduction

- Pain is the most common symptom arising in the mouth, face and neck and is the most common reason for emergency patient attendance to a dental surgery.
- The biological value of pain is that it usually signifies tissue damage. However, the severity of pain is not always proportional to the extent of damage, and pain may occasionally arise in the absence of organic damage.
- Pain usually arises peripherally, by stimulation of receptors, and is modified centrally. Thus, the perception of pain may be complicated by cultural, cognitive (e.g. attention, distraction) and emotional factors and modified by previous painful experiences.

Diagnosis of pain

- Pain is a subjective symptom and unlike an ulcer, there may be nothing to assess visually. The history is, therefore, paramount.
- A complaint of pain is clarified by the following 12 questions:
  1. How would you describe the pain? (adjectives such as sharp/stabbing or dull/throbbing are often forthcoming.)
  2. Where is the pain most severe? (the patient should be asked to point to the site of maximum intensity.)
  3. Where does the pain spread to? (the patient should outline the area with a finger.)
  4. How severe is the pain? (see pages 6, 73.)
  5. Does the pain prevent you getting to sleep or wake you up at night?
  6. When did the pain start?
  7. Is the pain continuous or does it come and go?
  8. If it comes and goes, how long does it last for each time?
  9. Does anything cause the pain to start?
  10. Does anything make the pain worse?
  11. Does anything make the pain better?
  12. Are there any other problems?

Many diagnostic pointers may be elicited from the history:

a. Character of the pain

Three characters of pain are commonly described:
Sharp/stabbing
Dull/throbbing/boring
Burning

Sharp/stabbing pain is often associated with:
Exposed dentine (sensitive root dentine, fractured restoration, fractured tooth, caries, cracked tooth)
Early pulpitis
Trigeminal neuralgia
Glossopharyngeal neuralgia

Dull/throbbing/boring pain is often associated with:
Late pulpitis
Apical and lateral periodontitis
Periodontal-endodontic lesion
Pericoronitis
Acute necrotizing ulcerative gingivitis (ANUG)
Dry socket
Periodic migrainous neuralgia
Herpes zoster
Giant cell arteritis
Tumours
Sinusitis
Temporomandibular joint disorders
Atypical odontalgia
Atypical facial pain

Burning pain is often associated with:
Burning mouth syndrome
Post-herpetic neuralgia
Ramsay Hunt syndrome

b. Severity of pain

- Severity of pain may be assessed by the patient scoring the pain on a scale of 0 to 10. Zero representing no pain and 10 representing the worst imaginable pain.
- If the patient has not resorted to analgesics, the pain may often not be severe. Pain controlled by mild analgesics such as aspirin is not severe.
- Pain preventing sleep or waking the sufferer up at night is often severe. Interestingly, atypical facial pain and trigeminal neuralgia, despite being unbearable during the day, do not affect sleep.

Periodic migrainous neuralgia characteristically disturbs sleep often at similar times of the night ('alarm clock awakening').

Acute pulpitis and acute periodontitis may prevent sleep and awaken a patient at night.

- Extreme (unbearable) pain, that may even lead to suicidal depression, may be associated with neuralgias such as:

Trigeminal neuralgia
Glossopharyngeal neuralgia
Periodic migrainous neuralgia
Post-herpetic neuralgia

c. Site of pain

- Pain arising from pathology is usually unilateral.
- Bilateral pain or pain crossing the midline may suggest:
  Sinusitis (if maxillary)
  Central nervous system disease
  Psychosomatic pain, e.g. atypical facial pain, atypical odontalgia, burning mouth syndrome.

d. Duration of pain

- Sharp stabbing pain usually lasts for a few seconds or minutes.
- Dull throbbing pain may last for hours, days or weeks.
- Pain is not usually continuous over very long periods of time. Continuous pain for years may suggest a psychosomatic origin.

e. Timing/exacerbating factors

- Excruciating pain on the merest contact with a trigger zone on the face suggests trigeminal neuralgia. Similar pain on swallowing suggests glossopharyngeal neuralgia.
- Pain on biting or touching a tooth may indicate acute periodontitis, or pericoronitis.
- Pain on hot or cold stimulation of a tooth suggests:
  Exposure of root or coronal dentine
  Caries
  Defective restoration
  Unlined recent restoration
  Cracked/fractured tooth
  Pulpitis
- Pain with sweet foods suggests:
  Exposure of root or coronal dentine (i.e. dentinal hypersensitivity)
  Caries
- Intermittent pain on biting, particularly on release of pressure, suggests a cracked tooth.
- Alcohol may precipitate periodic migrainous neuralgia.
- Pain related to meals may indicate:
  Salivary gland obstruction (salivary stimulation)

Temporomandibular joint disorder (pain with jaw movement)
Glossopharyngeal neuralgia (trigger zone in throat)
Trigeminal neuralgia (trigger zone on face)
Giant cell arteritis (muscle ischaemia—'masseteric claudication')
Dental or oral mucosal disease

f. Relieving factors

- Sharp/stabbing pains respond poorly to analgesics.
- Dull/throbbing pains usually respond to analgesics.
- Constant dull/throbbing pains of very long duration (years), completely unaffected by analgesics, may suggest atypical facial pain, atypical odontalgia or burning mouth syndrome.

g. Other symptoms

- Swelling, discharge, bad taste, bad breath, raised temperature, malaise or cervical lymphadenopathy may indicate an infective origin.

Try to identify:

1. The nerve, division and branch involved:

Usually the trigeminal nerve is involved, however, at the angle of the mandible the great auricular nerve may be involved (Fig. 5.1).

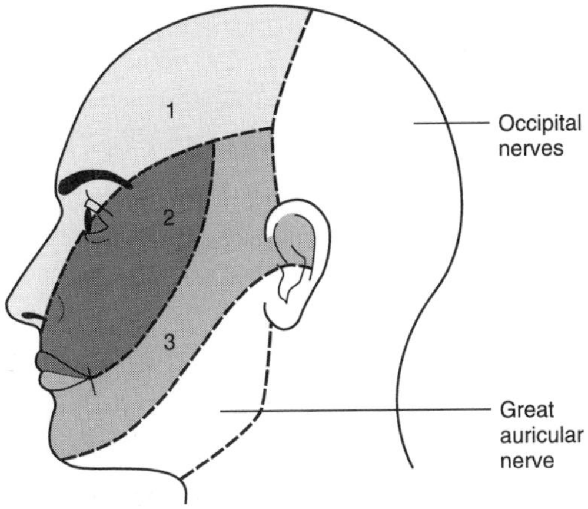

Figure 5.1 Sensory distribution of the trigeminal nerve; 1. Ophthalmic branch; 2. Maxillary branch; 3. Mandibular branch.

In the region of the posterior tongue and throat, the glossopharyngeal nerve may be implicated.

2. Likely site of cause of pain:

Peripheral — one branch involved, only.
Proximal — more than one branch involved.
Intracranial — more than one division involved and possible signs of raised intracranial pressure:
Severe headache
Vomiting
Clouding of consciousness
Unresponsive, dilated pupil on affected side

Pain may be dental or non-dental in origin, the symptoms of which may be similar and thus lead to diagnostic problems.

Pain of dental origin

Pain of dental origin is usually:
- Unilateral (unless both sides of the arch are involved).
- Never referred across to the other side of the face (except in the incisor region where some decussation of fibres across the midline may occur).
- Periodontal pain (acute periodontitis, pericoronitis) is usually well localized and the patient can point to the tooth involved.
- Pulpal pain is poorly localized and may be referred to another tooth on the same side of the arch, the opposite arch on the same side (usually the same relative position, i.e. upper 5 to lower 5 region). Occasionally, pain may be referred to any tissues supplied by any branch of the trigeminal nerve on the same side.
- The commonest source of pain in the region of the jaws is the dental pulp.
- Since common things occur commonly, eliminate them first!
- A diagnostic local anaesthetic injection may help to locate the arch and region from which pain is arising.

1. Pulpal pain

Dentine sensitivity
- Caused by dentine exposure and opening of dentine tubules:

Caries, tooth fracture (see 'cracked cusp', below), lost, fractured or marginally defective restoration, cement lute loss/failure, gingival recession, attrition, abrasion and erosion. Placement of a recent, unlined, metal restoration may lead to pain on application of hot and cold stimuli.

MH. e.g. Gastric reflux as a result of hiatus hernia, eating disorder or alcoholism (gastric acid erosion leading to opening of dentine tubules).

DH. e.g. Recent dental scaling, recent restorations, gingival recession, etc.

SH. e.g. High acid diet (dietary acid causing opening of dentine tubules).

Symptoms

- Sharp stabbing 'nerve' type pain, always related to a hot, cold or sweet stimulus; the pain is never spontaneous (i.e. a stimulus is always needed).
- Pain occurs immediately following application of the stimulus and is reasonably well localized (the patient can point to the area and often the tooth involved).
- Immediate relief follows removal of the stimulus.

(Note the similarity to early reversible pulpitis, described below.)

Note: Pain resulting from dentine caries may also be produced for 10 to 20 minutes after ingestion of a sugary meal. This is a result of local acid production by plaque bacteria.

Signs

- May include:
  Gingival recession.
  Caries, fractured or leaking restoration.
  Bubbles of saliva when moving a bridge retainer, indicating lute failure.
  Tooth wear/tooth surface loss (attrition, abrasion, erosion).

Diagnostic tests

- Identify the offending tooth/teeth by cold air, ethyl chloride or hot gutta percha, after isolating individual teeth using cotton rolls.

Treatment

- Depends on the cause:
  Treat caries/fractures/defective restorations.

  For sensitive root dentine, eliminate the cause, e.g. dietary acid. The patient may apply Sensodyne F® toothpaste on a brush and burnish it into the tooth surface, using a finger. A fluoride mouthrinse (0.05%) should be used daily, last thing at night.

Cracked tooth

- Cracks may involve:
  Enamel only (usually symptomless)
  Enamel and dentine only
  Enamel, dentine and pulp
  Root
  Crown and root

Fractures may be single or multiple.

Cracks involving enamel and dentine but not pulp:

- This may prove a puzzling and frustrating condition for both patient and dentist.
- Cracks usually result from an unexpected encounter with a hard object (e.g. cherry stone, bone) during mastication, or a blow to the chin.
- Mandibular 1st molar teeth are most commonly affected, followed by mandibular 2nd molars, maxillary 1st molars, and maxillary premolars, in descending order.
- Both genders are affected equally, and patients are usually middle-aged.

MH. There are no medical disorders that predispose to cracked teeth.

DH. The periodontal status of affected patients is usually good, there being no tooth mobility, and an opposing natural tooth is present. A well supported tooth and opponent are required to generate sufficient force to crack the tooth. The affected tooth may also have a large restoration without cuspal coverage.

Symptoms

- Can be varied and may lead to misdiagnosis.
- Occasional sharp pain on biting foods of a firm consistency on a certain area of a tooth. The conditions that produce the pain are often unique, and therefore difficult to reproduce in the dental surgery.
- Pain is intermittent and may be worse on relief of a biting force than on application of the force. This is known as 'rebound pain' and is due to dentine surfaces rubbing together, causing tubular fluid movement.
- The pain is well localized and does not usually refer.
- Pain is of very short duration, limited to biting and never spontaneous.
- There may also be some sensitivity to heat and (especially) cold, due to stimulation of the pulp via the fracture line.

- Patients may not seek treatment for a considerable time since the problem occurs only intermittently.

> *Keywords*
> Intermittent, occasional pain on biting
> Well localized
> Rebound pain
> Vital tooth

Signs

- In order to allow transmission of sufficient load to crack a tooth, an opposing natural tooth is usually present and the periodontal status of the affected and opposing teeth is usually excellent.
- Non-adhesive restorations weaken a tooth and it is common to find cracked teeth with MOD restorations, especially amalgam or non cusp-covered inlays. Similarly, deep developmental fissures extending through a cusp or marginal ridge, and the canine fossa of maxillary first premolars may be implicated.
- The crack may be visible, especially if stained.

Diagnostic tests

- Use light reflected from a mouth mirror onto the tooth at different angles, fibre optic transillumination and magnification to visualize the crack.
- Biting on cotton wool, a wooden spatula, rubber dam or a rubber polishing wheel may allow the crack to open, cause pain and thus allow the affected tooth to be indentified. Painting the tooth beforehand with a dye such as methylene blue or washable ink may allow entry of the dye into the opened crack. The dye will remain in the crack when the tooth is cleaned.
- The radiographic appearance will be normal; fine cracks cannot be visualized on a radiograph.

Treatment

- Remove any associated restoration and investigate the extent of the fracture line.
- Adjust the occlusion to reduce loading of the offending cusp.
- Placement of adhesive restorations, such as glass ionomer cements, composite resins and bonded amalgam may be effective in preventing propagation of the fracture in the short term. However, they are often ineffective, by themselves, in the long term.
- Placement of a full veneer crown or adhesive metal onlay to splint the remaining tooth structure is more effective. As an

emergency measure, the tooth may be modestly reduced, to allow placement of a temporary aluminium (or similar) crown form. Orthodontic bands and copper rings are (less satisfactory) alternatives.
- Definitive restoration should be delayed until the pulpal condition has been determined. If root canal therapy is required, this can be undertaken through the temporary crown.

Cracked tooth involving the pulp

Symptoms
- May start with the same aforementioned symptoms but will progress to pulpal inflammation (see below). This may result in spontaneous pain referred throughout the divisions of the trigeminal nerve, causing extreme diagnostic difficulties.
- The pulpitis passes through initial (hyperaemia/reversible), acute (irreversible) and suppurative stages, leading to severe persistant throbbing pain.
- Temporary relief may follow pulp death, only to be followed by acute apical periodontitis, when the tooth becomes tender to percussion and is easily localized.

Diagnostic tests
- As above, include vitality tests.
- Radiographs may show widening of the periodontal ligament space.

Treatment
- If the tooth can be saved, root canal treat after exploration of the fracture line and splinting with a temporary crown form.
- Occasionally, hemisection or premolarization may be indicated.

Pulpitis

Classification:

Initial pulpitis (hyperaemia)
Acute pulpitis
Suppurative pulpitis (pulpal abscess)
Chronic pulpitis
Chronic hyperplastic pulpitis (pulp polyp)

Initial pulpitis (hyperaemia of the pulp)
MH. Nil.

DH. e.g. Recent dental scaling (lateral canals), recent/deep restoration, deep caries, history of trauma, etc.

Symptoms

- Unilateral, sharp, stabbing pain, recognized as a 'toothache'.
- The pain is intermittent and of immediate onset to hot, cold and sweet stimuli.
- The tooth is not painful unless stimulated and may respond more to cold than hot stimuli.
- The pain on stimulation is of very short duration; it does not linger for more than 10 to 15 seconds after the stimulus has been removed.
- The painful tooth is difficult to localize. The patient may be unable to point to the offending tooth.

> *Keywords*
> Pain only on stimulation
> Disappears on removal of stimulus
> Very short duration (less than 15 seconds)
> No spontaneous pain
> Poorly localized

Signs

- May include a large intracoronal or extracoronal restoration, large carious lesion involving the pulp, or a pin placed close to, or involving, the pulp.

Diagnostic tests

- Percussion: No tenderness or dullness to percussion.
- Vitality tests: The offending tooth gives an exaggerated response to vitality tests, in comparison to normal adjacent teeth.
- The tooth is of normal colour.
- Radiographs: Will detail caries and/or dental restorations. Normal radiographic appearance of apical and periodontal tissues. No loss of apical lamina dura, no apical radiolucency.

Treatment

- Remove the cause (e.g. caries), dress deep cavities using a calcium hydroxide lining and sedative temporary filling, e.g. zinc oxide/eugenol cement. The initial pulpitis may sometimes be reversed if the cause is eliminated.
- Review; if symptoms abate, the pulp may have recovered or died. Repeat vitality tests are, therefore, essential.
- Serial radiographs (3, 6 and 12 months) are also required to monitor the apical condition and identify any sclerosis of the canal that may result from low grade chronic pulpal inflammation. Endodontics will be required if early sclerosis is

identified. If endodontics is delayed, the canal may be obstructed and root treatment may prove impossible.

Acute pulpitis

This condition is usually irreversible and may lead on to suppurative pulpitis (pulpal abscess).

MH. Nil.

DH. Large restoration/caries lesion, history of dental trauma, etc., as detailed above.

Symptoms

- Unilateral, initially sharp and stabbing pain, becoming dull or throbbing with time. The sharp, stabbing pain is often interspersed with periods of a dull ache.
- Initially, the pain is an exaggerated response to mainly hot stimuli, and is of long duration, persisting for more than 15 seconds (even up to several hours) after the stimulus is removed.
- Radiation of pain is widespread and referral is common.
- As the condition developes, pain occurs spontaneously (i.e. without an obvious stimulus) and is often worse at night.
- Pain may prevent sleep or awaken the patient from sleep.
- Since the pain is due to increased pulpal pressure, lying down or bending increases the pressure and thus the pain.
- Cold may reduce pressure and provide temporary relief.
- Problems persist for several days or weeks and then stop quite suddenly as the pulp necroses.
- The pain is poorly localized until the tooth becomes tender to bite on, following pulp death, as an acute apical periodontitis develops.

> *Keywords*
> Pain persists after removal of stimulus
> Spontaneous pain
> Poorly localized
> Exaggerated result to heat and electrical vitality test
> Cold may reduce pain

Signs

- Large restoration/carious lesion, fractured or discoloured tooth, etc.
- The tooth will initially not be tender to bite on, but will become tender in the late stages as apical periodontitis develops.

Diagnostic tests
- A diagnostic local anaesthetic may be required to localize the affected tooth, as may diagnostic removal of restorations and caries to examine for pulpal exposure, deep caries, fractures, etc.
- Initially, there will be an exaggerated response to heat and electrical vitality tests. Later, there will be no response, as the pulp dies. Cold may relieve pain by reducing pulpal pressure.
- Vitality test results may be confusing in multirooted teeth since one root may contain vital tissue and another necrotic material.
- In later stages, the tooth may become tender to percussion and provide a dull percussive note as apical periodontitis develops.
- Radiographs: May reveal deep caries/restoration, etc., widening of the periodontal ligament space and in the late stages loss of apical lamina dura.

Treatment
- Eliminate the cause (e.g. caries), then consider endodontics or extraction of the affected tooth.

Chronic pulpitis

MH. Nil.
DH. Large restoration, etc., as above.

Symptoms
- Intermittent, mild pain over a long period (months or years).
- The pain is poorly localized and may be limited to occasional hypersensitivity to heat.
- Painful symptoms of chronic pulpitis are rarely the patients main concern but may be described as an incidental matter.

Signs
- Large restoration, etc., as detailed above.

Diagnostic tests
- Vitality: A gradual reaction, leading to an exaggerated response to heat is common. The response to cold and electrical tests is reduced, in comparison to healthy, vital teeth.
- There may be very minor tenderness and dullness to percussion.
- Radiographs: May reveal sclerosis of the pulp chamber and root canal, and some loss of lamina dura, apically. The alveolar bone in the region of the root apex may also be sclerosed.

Treatment
- Endodontics or extraction. Root canal treatment of sclerosed canals may prove difficult and occasionally impossible.

Chronic hyperplastic pulpitis (pulp polyp)
MH. Nil.
DH. Usually dental neglect in a young patient.

Symptoms
- Usually none, although the patient may complain of a lump in the mouth.

Signs
- Visible pulp polyp within a grossly carious tooth.
- Extensive carious destruction of coronal tooth tissue is usual.

Diagnostic tests
- Radiographs will confirm the extent of the coronal caries. The apical foramina will be large, allowing the excellent pulpal blood flow required for this condition to occur.

Treatment
- Extraction.

Galvanism
- Caused by production of an electrical current, due to approximation of dissimilar metals in the presence of an electrolyte (saliva).

MH. Nil.

DH. Recent metallic restoration, adjacent to, or opposing, another metallic restoration.

Symptoms
- Intermittent pain, similar to that experienced by many when biting on silver paper.
- Pain occurs only after placement of a new metal restoration, is well localized and does not refer.

Signs
- Recent metallic restoration abutting or opposing an existing metallic restoration.
- Corrosion deposits or damage may be evident.

Treatment
- Reassure that the problem will diminish over a few days, as corrosion products accumulate.

- If severe, apply a temporary coat of resin or varnish over the new restoration.

Aerodontalgia
- Dental pain occurring only at reduced atmospheric pressure.

MH. Possible sinusitis.

DH. Recent restoration.

Symptoms
- Acute pulpitic pain (see above), only during decompression or flying at high altitude.

Signs
- Recently restored teeth (suggesting minor pulpitis).
- Aerosinusitis may be a contributing factor if maxillary teeth are involved.

Diagnostic tests
- Radiographs: Possible antral opacity on panoral radiograph (sinusitis). Dental radiographs may show a deep restoration. No apical pathology will be seen.

Treatment
- Monitor; the pulpitis might prove to be reversible or irreversible. If irreversible, root canal treat or extract.
- Refer for investigation and treatment of any sinusitis.

2. Periodontal pain

Acute apical periodontitis of pulpal origin
- The source of the apical infection is the pulp chamber.

MH. Nil.

DH. Possible history of severe trauma to teeth, or large restoration/carious cavity, pins near or into the pulp or defective endodontics. There is usually a history of prior toothache (acute pulpitis). However, the tooth will (usually) be no longer sensitive to heat or cold.

Symptoms
- Unilateral, severe, continuous, dull/throbbing pain, of very rapid onset.
- The tooth is exquisitely tender to touch and biting, and may feel ‘high’ in the bite. The tooth may also feel loose.

- Pain is severe enough to prevent eating and sleep and may awaken the patient at night.
- Pain is very well localized; the patient will always be able to point to the offending tooth and may try to protect the tooth from the touch or mirror handle of the investigating dentist.
- Soft tissue swelling may also be associated, usually soft and puffy (collateral oedema — differentiate from the brawny swelling of cellulitis).
- Pain is often reduced as the swelling appears or an abscess points, due to release of pressure.
- Painful swelling of the face, buccal sulcus, palate or neck (see below) may be reported, and the patient looks and feels unwell.
- If posterior teeth are involved, the patient may be unable to open their mouth fully, while involvement of the upper anterior teeth may lead to facial swelling and eye closure.

Keywords
Very well localized
Tooth exquisitely tender to pressure
Tooth feels 'high' in the bite
Negative vitality test response

Signs

- Large restorations/caries/pins/defective root canal filling etc.
- Surrounding gingival tissues may be inflamed.
- If there is discharge of pus through the gingival crevice, a pocket may be present.
- The regional lymph nodes are often enlarged and tender.
- The patient may be pyrexic and malaised.
- The offending tooth may be discoloured (pulpal bleeding into dentine tubules).
- There may be soft tissue swelling in the region of the apex buccally or labially and/or a sinus.
- The tooth will be extruded and mobile.
- Palpation of any soft tissue swelling may reveal that it is:
  Soft — local oedema
  Firm (brawny) and erythematous — cellulitis

Diagnostic tests

- Percussion: The tooth will be mobile and exquisitely tender to percussion. Tenderness is particularly to pressure applied in an apical direction. The percussion note will be dull (indicating fluid accumulation in the periodontal ligament).
- Vitality tests: Will usually be negative but occasionally are

unreliable — pus may conduct the stimulus, or the tooth may be multi-rooted with some remaining vital tissue in one or more canals. The tooth may respond to heat as a result of expansion of gases in the pulp chamber. Cold may relieve pain by reducing pressure within the pulp chamber and apical tissues.
- Radiology: Initially widening of the periodontal ligament space with loss of definition of the lamina dura. Followed by increasing periapical radiolucency. Radiological signs may be delayed.

Treatment
- Open and drain if pus is accumulating (do not leave teeth open for longer than overnight). Incision and drainage of any pus in soft tissues is essential. Open, clean and dress the root canal.
- Submucosal infiltration (0.1–0.2 ml) local anaesthesia, after use of topical anaesthetic, may allow incision and drainage to be carried out. However, infiltration into a site of infection may be ineffective and lead to spread of infection. Wherever possible regional anaesthesia should be employed to ensure effective pain relief.
- Antibiotics may be required if drainage or extraction have to be delayed or systemic symptoms are present. Antibiotics do not eliminate the need for establishing drainage.
- Endodontics or extraction after acute inflammation has been treated.

Note: A so-called ‘Phoenix’ abscess may arise as an acute inflammatory episode during endodontic therapy as a result of re-activation of existing infection, or re-infection of the root canal during treatment.

Traumatic periodontitis
- Inflammatory (not infective) periodontitis due to trauma, for example a recently placed ‘high’ restoration or excessive loading during orthodontic treatment or after the fitting of a partial denture.

MH. Nil.

DH. Recent restoration, inlay, crown, bridge or denture. Current orthodontic treatment, appliance recently fitted or adjusted.

Symptoms
- Well localized pain on biting or on application of pressure. The patient can identify the offending tooth, which will feel ‘high’ in the bite.
- The tooth may feel slightly loose.

Signs

- Recent restoration, which, if metallic, may show a burnish mark on the occlusal surface, indicating a premature contact.
- Presence of a new or recently modified orthodontic appliance or partial denture.
- The tooth may be slightly mobile.

Diagnostic tests

- Vitality: Unlike an infective periapical periodontitis, there will be a normal response to heat, cold, and electrical tests.
- Percussion: Minor tenderness to percussion and a dull percussion note, due to traumatic inflammation of the periodontal ligament.
- Identify occlusal contacts using articulating paper.

Keywords
Symptoms similar to acute (infective) apical periodontitis
But tooth is vital

Treatment

- Occlusal adjustment of any implicated restoration.
- Adjust orthodontic appliance or denture, or if necessary refer back to orthodontist/prosthetist.

Chronic apical periodontitis (apical granuloma)

MH. Nil.

DH. Large restoration, pins, defective root canal filling, etc. (see Acute apical periodontitis, above).

Symptoms

- Pain is unusual, but when it occurs is dull and throbbing and not well localized.
- There may be an occasional discharge (bad taste) if a sinus is present.

Signs

- Large restoration, etc., the tooth may be discoloured and a sinus may be present.

Diagnostic tests

- Percussion: Possible minor tenderness to percussion and a slightly dull percussion note.
- Vitality: Usually negative. Heat may occasionally cause a response by expansion of gases in the pulp chamber.

- Radiographs: An apical radiolucency will be present, which may be large and well defined. A previous, inadequate, root canal filling or pulp dressing may be evident.
- A gutta percha point passed along any sinus track will pass to the apex of the affected tooth and will be visible on a radiograph. This is often a useful diagnostic tool.

Treatment

- Endodontics or extraction.
- Apical surgery is indicated only after conventional root treatment has been attempted and failed, or cannot be attempted (post and core present, etc.).

Tracking of pus

- Tracking of pus from periapical infection depends upon anatomical relationships (Fig. 5.2):

Posterior maxillary teeth — Pus tracks through the buccal plate, usually below the buccinator muscle attachment, Thus, pus often points intraorally, into the buccal sulcus.

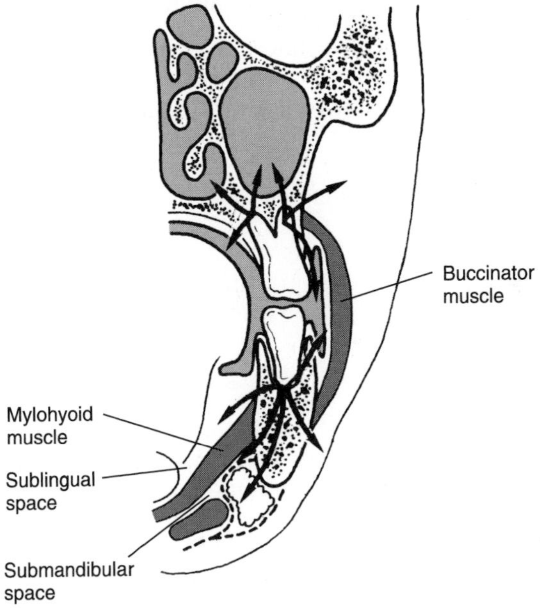

Figure 5.2 Directions in which pus from a periapical lesion may track (see text).

Occasionally, the apex of a root (e.g. upper canine or first molar apex) may be above the buccinator attachment. In this case, pus points extraorally, onto the face.

Palatal root of the maxillary first molar — This is sited palatally. Thus, pus often tracks into the palate. Due to their proximity, pus may also track to the floor of the antrum or (rarely) the nose.

Upper incisors (excluding the lateral incisor) — Pus tracks into the labial sulcus or, rarely, into the floor of the nose.

Upper lateral incisor — The apex of this tooth is directed palatally. In this case, pus points into the anterior palate.

Most lower teeth — The apices are above the buccinator muscle origin. Therefore, pus tracks intraorally into the buccal sulcus. However, with lower anterior teeth, the apices may be below the mentalis muscle attachment and pus may point on the chin.

Lower second and third molars — The apices of these teeth are closer to the lingual wall of the body of the mandible than the buccal wall. Therefore pus may track lingually. Since the apices are often below the attachment of the mylohyoid muscle, pus may pass into the submandibular space and may point on the neck.

Lower first molars — The apices may be below the buccinator muscle origin. Therefore, pus may point extraorally, onto the face.

(See also Pericoronitis, below.)

Acute periodontitis of gingival origin (lateral periodontal/parodontal abscess)

MH. More common in patients with diabetes mellitus or immunocompromised patients.
DH. History of gingival disease, abscess, tooth loss, tooth drifting/looseness, dental neglect.

Symptoms

- Well localized, continuous, dull and throbbing pain.
- The affected tooth, and possibly other teeth may be loose.
- A bad taste or smell will accompany any discharge into the mouth.
- There may be an associated painful swelling in the mouth.
- Extraoral swelling is very rare.
- The tooth may be painful on biting and may feel 'high' in the bite.

Signs
- Teeth will be mobile and deep pocketing will be present.
- Poor oral hygiene, plaque and calculus deposits.
- A sinus may be present or pus may be draining from the pocket.
- Inserting a periodontal pocket measuring probe down a pocket will release pus.
- Probing any sinus may lead to a deep pocket.
- The tooth may be in supra-occlusion.

Diagnostic tests
- Vitality: Unlike apical periodontitis of pulpal origin, vitality tests are positive (but see Periodontic-endodontic lesions, below).
- Percussion: Tenderness to percussion, particularly to lateral forces. The percussion note will be dull, due to accumulation of fluid in the periodontal ligament space.
- Radiographs: Will show generalized bone loss, with a horizontal and/or vertical pattern.

Keywords
Pain on biting/pressure
Mobile tooth/teeth
Deep pocketing
Positive vitality tests

Treatment
- Establish drainage through the pocket or by incision.
- Provide oral hygiene instruction, and advise hot salt water mouth rinses and chlorhexidine mouth rinse.
- Antibiotics are unnessary unless systemic upset is present.
- Treat the underlying periodontal disease.
- Unsavable teeth should be extracted after resolution of the acute phase.

Periodontal-endodontic lesions
- Molar teeth are most commonly involved; they possess most lateral and furcation canals.
- May be primarily periodontal in origin:
  i. Deep pocket to apex.
  ii. Recession or scaling instrumentation involving lateral/furcation canals.
- Or primarily endodontic in origin:
  i. Apical lesion tracking through the periodontal ligament to discharge through the gingival crevice.
  ii. Pulpal lesion tracking through a lateral canal.

iii. Root perforations during endodontic therapy or post and core preparation.
iv. Vertical root fracture.
v. Horizontal root fracture in communication with the gingival sulcus.

- Or truly coexisting, i.e. separate in aetiology but both present on the same tooth (unusual).
- Thus, an endodontic lesion may mimic a periodontal lesion, while a periodontal lesion may mimic an endodontic lesion. Alternatively, both lesions may coexist!

Signs and symptoms
- As for apical or lateral periodontitis (see above) or a combination, depending on the aetiology.

Diagnostic tests
- Vitality: No response if primarily endodontic or combined. Response if primarily periodontal.
- Percussion: Tenderness and a dull percussion note.
- Radiographs: Gutta percha point in pocket reaches apex.

Treatment
- Deep pocket to apex, pulp vital — Periodontal therapy.
- Deep pocket to apex, pulp non-vital — Root canal treatment plus periodontal therapy (commence endodontics first).
- Extract unsavable teeth.

3. Gingival pain

Traumatic gingivitis
- A localized gingival inflammation caused by physical (e.g. toothbrush, fish bone), chemical (e.g. aspirin burn) or electrical (rare) trauma.

Treatment
Includes reduction of the risk of any subsequent infection by use of hot salt water or chlorhexidine mouth rinses.

Acute necrotizing ulcerative gingivitis (ANUG)
- An infective disease, characterized by rapidly progressive ulceration of the interdental papillae.
- Ulceration starts at the tip of the papilla but spreads along the gingival margin and may lead to extensive destruction of the gingival tissues.

- Anaerobic Gram negative organisms are involved.
- It is probably an opportunistic infection where host resistance is reduced.
- Young to middle-aged adults are affected and the condition is possibly more common in males.
- It is uncommon in children and when thought to be present has usually been confused with herpetic gingivostomatitis.

MH. Smoker (reduced gingival blood flow), heavy drinker, psychological stress, upper respiratory tract infection, immunosuppression (including HIV disease).

DH. Irregular attender, neglected dentition, very poor plaque removal.

Symptoms

- Moderate to severe gingival tenderness, causing pain when eating and toothbrushing.
- Pain is dull/boring in character, is sometimes accompanied by bad breath (halitosis) and an unpleasant metallic taste.
- The gums bleed spontaneously.

Signs

- Usually dental neglect with obvious (often copious) plaque and calculus deposits. However, in the immunocompromised, ANUG may develop despite good oral hygiene.
- Oral malodour is marked and is caused by accumulation of products from anaerobic bacteria and necrotic tissue.
- The gingival margin is ulcerated with destruction of the interdental papilla often giving rise to a punched out crater.
- A grey pseudomembrane lies over the gingival tissues. Profuse bleeding occurs if the pseudomembrane is removed.
- The disease is limited to the gingival tissues; mucosal involvement only arises in profound malnutrition or immunosuppression.
- Pyrexia, malaise and cervical lymphadenopathy are uncommon features of ANUG.

Keywords
Usually very poor oral hygiene
Ulcerated interdental papillae
Immunosuppression

Diagnostic tests

- Gram negative organisms in smears.

- Blood tests are indicated if disease is severe, recurrent or accompanied by systemic upset, to exclude leukaemia and other causes of immunosuppression.

Treatment
- Debride and irrigate the tissues, as much as the patient will tolerate.
- Prescribe metronidazole 200 mg tds for five days and hydrogen peroxide mouth rinse (20 vols diluted 1:4) or chlorhexidine mouthwash.
- Provide oral hygiene instruction and undertake scaling and polishing after resolution of the acute phase.
- Reduce or avoid tobacco smoking.

Acute pericoronitis
- This is a bacterial infection of tissues around a partially erupted tooth. Communication with the mouth allows infection of the pocket around the unerupted component of the crown.
- Mandibular third molar teeth are most commonly involved.
- Trauma from a maxillary molar biting onto the operculum flap overlying the mandibular tooth is a major contributing factor.

MH. Psychological stress and upper respiratory tract infections may predispose. The condition is most common in autumn and spring and possibly during university/college examinations.

DH. Presence of partially erupted lower third molar—rarely with other erupting permanent teeth. Therefore, the maximum incidence is around 20 years of age.

Symptoms
- Dull throbbing pain, well localized to the region of the lower third molar tooth. The patient can point to the offending area.
- Swelling may occur over and beneath the angle of the mandible.
- There may be difficulty in opening the mouth and pain on swallowing.
- The patient feels generally unwell.
- Neck and jaw pain may be present if the cervical or submandibular lymph nodes are affected.

Signs
- Trismus; intraoral examination is often very difficult.
- Intraoral swelling may extend to the angle of the mandible.

- Extraorally there may be a tender submandibular and upper cervical lymphadenopathy.
- The operculum flap and gingival tissue in the area of the third molar is swollen and beads of pus may be evident under the operculum flap.
- The upper wisdom tooth occludes onto the inflammed operculum.
- Pyrexia may be present.

Keywords
Well localized pain
Partially erupted wisdom tooth
Opposing tooth biting on operculum flap

Diagnostic tests
- The third molar, if not visible, will be palpable to probing (i.e. in communication with mouth). Completely unerupted teeth, with no communication with the mouth, do not cause pain.
- Lymph node examination: cervical lymphadenopathy will often be found.
- Radiographs: The partially erupted wisdom tooth will be evident often with an enlarged follicle space around the crown.

Treatment
- Grind the maxillary wisdom tooth cusps out of contact with the operculum flap, or extract the upper wisdom tooth.
- Irrigate under the flap with warm saline, chlorhexidine mouthwash or gel.
- Antibiotics, typically metronidazole or penicillin V, should be prescribed if lymphadenopathy or systemic upset are present.
- Hot salt water mouthrinses may be used every 2 hours.
- Analgesics may be used, if required.
- Extract the lower third molar (if required) only after resolution of the acute phase, due to the risk of spread of infection and dry socket.

Tracking of pus from third molar infection (Fig. 5.3)
Pus may track into the peritonsillar space, the lateral pharyngeal space, the pterygoid space, or track into the mandibular buccal sulcus. Alternatively, pus may penetrate the buccinator muscle laterally, to enter the parotid space or discharge onto the face.

Migratory abscess of the buccal sulcus
Occasionally, pus tracks submucosally from the third molar

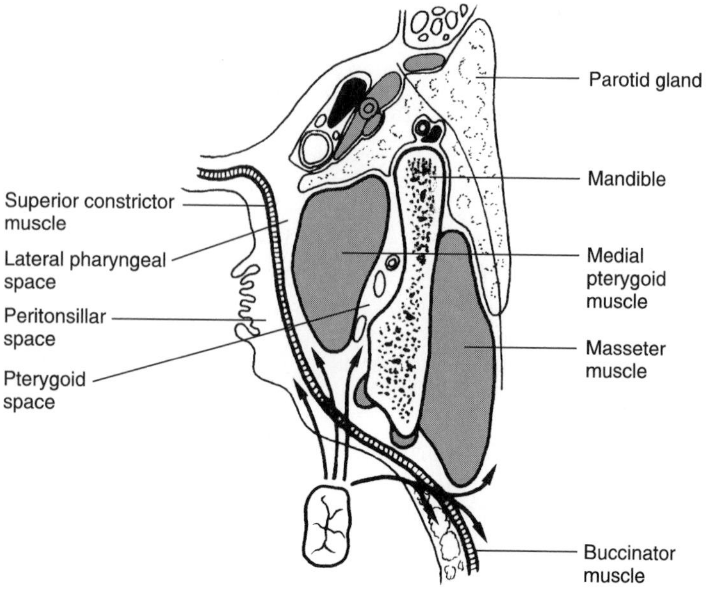

Figure 5.3 Tracking of pus from third molar infection.

region, along the gutter formed between the body of the mandible and the external oblique ridge, and presents in the buccal sulcus adjacent to the first molar tooth. Where treatment has been delayed, an intraoral sinus may be present.

Teething

- A pericoronitis around erupting (usually primary) teeth.

MH. Possible coincidence with a viral infection.

- This condition is self limiting and does not usually require treatment. If severe, an analgesic gel (e.g. lignocaine) may be useful.

'Desquamative' gingivitis

- The term 'desquamative' is descriptive only and does not constitute a diagnosis. It is used where the gingivae appear red or raw.
- Causes include lichen planus (see pages 205, 220) and mucous membrane pemphigoid (see page 202).
- Diagnosis of the cause should be confirmed by biopsy.

4. Bone pain

Dry socket

- The most common complication of tooth extraction.
- Reduced blood supply, infection and trauma during extraction are predisposing factors.

MH. Possible radiotherapy to jaws, Paget's disease.

DH. Recent extraction, usually of a lower molar tooth, especially an impacted wisdom tooth, 2–4 days previously. Dry sockets rarely affect the upper arch.

Symptoms

- Dull, throbbing, continuous, severe, deep seated 'bone' pain in the area of the extraction, often accompanied by bad breath.
- Pain arising a few days after extraction is usually due to formation of a dry socket.
- The extraction site is painful to touch and when eating.

Signs

- Oral malodour is common.
- Examination of the socket reveals that the clot has been destroyed and the socket is empty or contains debris.
- The gingiva around the socket is red and inflamed.
- When the debris is washed away, whitish dead bone may be visible lining the socket.

Keywords
Bone pain a few days after extraction

Treatment

- Remove debris and irrigate the socket with warm normal saline.
- Dress with Alvogyl® in the socket.
- Warn the patient that pain may persist for 1 week.
- Analgesics may be required.

Osteomyelitis
See Chapter 8.

Infected Dental Cyst
See Chapter 9.

Trauma, Fracture
See Chapter 7.

5. Pain associated with denture bases

- This may be due to ill-fitting or overextended bases, occlusal errors, pressure on bony projections or nerves (e.g. mental nerve) and teeth or roots erupting under the denture base.

Symptoms
- Pain when eating.

Signs
- Pain with pressure on the denture teeth in the region of the problem, erythema or ulceration of mucosa at the border of the denture, roots or teeth beneath the denture base, sharp alveolar ridge.

Treatment
- Eliminate the cause.

Further reading

Fox, K. and Youngson, C. (1997) Diagnosis and treatment of the cracked tooth. *Primary Dental Care,* **4**, 109–113.

Juniper, R.P. and Parkins, B.J. (1990) *Emergencies in Dental Practice: Diagnosis and Management.* Oxford: Butterworth-Heinemann.

6

Pain of non-dental origin

Summary

Differential diagnosis

1. **Neurologic**
   Trigeminal neuralgia
   Glossopharyngeal neuralgia
   Herpes zoster
   Post-herpetic neuralgia
   Geniculate herpes (Ramsay–Hunt syndrome)
   Bell's palsy
   Multiple sclerosis
   HIV disease (see Chapters 8 and 10)
   Intracranial tumours
   Causalgia
2. **Vascular origin**
   Migraine
   Periodic migrainous neuralgia
   Paroxysmal facial hemicrania
   Giant cell arteritis
   Referred pain, e.g. cardiac ischaemia
3. **Maxillary antrum/nasopharynx**
   Sinusitis
   Malignancy
4. **Salivary glands**
   Acute bacterial sialadentitis (see Chapter 12)
   Chronic bacterial sialadentitis (see Chapter 12)
   Sjögren's syndrome (see Chapter 13)
   Malignancy (see Chapters 10 and 12)
   Calculi, stenosis of duct, obstruction of duct orifice
   HIV disease (see Chapter 12)
   Mumps (see Chapter 8)
5. **Oral mucosa**
   Herpes zoster (see above)
   Geniculate herpes (Ramsay–Hunt syndrome) (see above)
   Herpetic gingivostomatitis (see Chapter 10)
   Late stage carcinoma (see Chapters 10 and 12)
   Mucosal ulceration (see Chapter 10)

continued

6. **Jaws/masticatory muscles**
   Temporomandibular joint disorders
   Fractures (see Chapter 7)
   Osteomyelitis (see Chapter 8)
   Infected cysts (see Chapter 9)
   Malignancy (see Chapter 12)
7. **Ears**
   Otitis media
8. **Eyes**
   Glaucoma
9. **Psychogenic**
   Atypical facial pain
   Atypical odontalgia
   Burning mouth syndrome

(See Chapter 5 for Introduction to Pain.)

- Pain of non-dental origin is less common than pain of dental origin.
- The most common causes of pain of non-dental origin are the temporomandibular joint disorders.

1. Neurologic

Trigeminal neuralgia

- Sudden, very severe, brief (seconds only), recurrent stabbing pain in the distribution of the trigeminal nerve (see Fig. 5.1).
- It is a rare condition, mainly limited to the middle-aged and elderly.
- In affected patients under 40 years, suspect serious underlying pathology, e.g. tumour or multiple sclerosis. Approximately 3% of patients presenting with trigeminal neuralgia have multiple sclerosis.
- All patients with trigeminal neuralgia must undergo a detailed neurological examination, particularly of the cranial nerves (see Chapter 4).
- Trigeminal neuralgia is up to twice more common in women.
- The right side is affected more than the left (1.7:1).
- Very rarely (4%) pain may occur bilaterally.

Aetiologies include
Demyelination
Vascular compression of the trigeminal ganglion
Trauma or infection of the nerve
Idiopathic

MH. Association with multiple sclerosis.

Symptoms
(Diagnosis is made by the history).

- Unilateral, shortlasting (seconds) excruciating, unbearable, stabbing (lancinating), paroxysmal face pain, affecting a predictable site.
- There are few more painful conditions.

The characteristics of the pain are:

- Pain is typically limited to one of the three divisions of the trigeminal nerve, most commonly the 2nd and 3rd divisions.
- A trigger zone may be present somewhere along the distribution of the trigeminal nerve. The trigger zone may be refractory between paroxysms. Only light pressure on the trigger zone will induce severe pain. The patient may not shave or touch the face in the region of the trigger zone, for fear of inducing a paroxysm. Speech and swallowing may be limited if the trigger zone involves the mouth. Any neurological finding other than the presence of a trigger zone puts the diagnosis of trigeminal neuralgia in serious doubt.
- The pain of trigeminal neuralgia never crosses the midline and does not usually cross from one division to another in the same bout.
- Pain is described as sharp and stabbing, 'electric shock'/'red hot needle' type. It is of rapid onset, short duration and with rapid recovery. A series of jabs occur over several minutes. This is often followed by a dull ache which may last for several hours. Paroxysms occur most commonly in the first hours after awakening.
- The pain of trigeminal neuralgia clusters, patients having periods of daily pain, then periods of remission. The remission may last days, weeks, months or years.
- Of diagnostic significance, trigeminal neuralgia does not affect sleep.

Signs

- Tic douloureux (spasmodic contraction of face muscles due to the pain of trigeminal neuralgia).

Keywords
Very brief
Severe
Lancinating pain
Trigger zone
Trigeminal nerve distribution
Sleep not affected

Differential diagnosis
Neuropathy (due to a lesion pressing on the trigeminal nerve)
Herpes zoster (cutaneous lesions are diagnostic)
Atypical facial pain
Migrainous neuralgia
Pulpitis
Apical periodontitis

Treatment
- Refer for specialist oral medical/neurological care. Carbamazepine and/or phenytoin may be used. Cryotherapy, surgical section, thermocoagulation of peripheral nerve as it exits from the foramen may be attempted if pain is uncontrolled.

Pretrigeminal neuralgia
- May be reported by up to 20% of sufferers of trigeminal neuralgia.
- Presents as a mild toothache type pain in the absence of any other dental signs.
- Goes on to deteriorate into trigeminal neuralgia.

Glossopharyngeal neuralgia
- Much less common than trigeminal neuralgia.
- Middle-aged and the elderly are mainly affected.
- Underlying pathology (especially multiple sclerosis) must be excluded.

MH. Possible multiple myeloma, multiple sclerosis.

Symptoms
- Pain is identical to that of trigeminal neuralgia but affecting the glossopharyngeal rather than the trigeminal nerve.
- Two distributions of pain are recognized:
  1. Otic (pain related to the ear).
  2. Pharyngeal (pain related to the angle of the jaw, throat and neck).

- The trigger zone is located in the oropharynx and paroxysms may be initiated by swallowing.

Signs
- Vagal features sometimes occur (e.g. nausea, bradycardia) during paroxysms.

Treatment
- Refer for specialist care.

Herpes zoster (shingles)

- The only non-dental pain that may truly mimic pulpal pain (see Chapter 5).
- Zoster is a viral inflammation of a posterior root ganglion, affecting one or two peripheral sensory nerves.
- Herpes zoster causes chicken pox in children but (like herpes simplex) remains dormant in sensory ganglia until reactivated.
- Reactivation in adults gives rise to shingles.
- The disease is common but mainly limited to adults, often over 60 years old.
- In the trigeminal region the ophthalmic division is most commonly affected.
- The patient may present to the dentist if the 2nd or 3rd division of the trigeminal nerve is involved.

MH: Shingles can occur in otherwise well elderly persons. In young adults and children, immunosupression (e.g. HIV disease) can underly shingles, especially when severe and/or recurrent.

Symptoms
- Severe, unilateral, deep seated, burning pain, in the prodromal phase, a few days before the rash and vesicles develop.
- The vesicles become weeping and crusting on the skin but remain as shallow ulcers in the mouth. The vesicles and ulcers are typically unilateral in distribution.
- The patient will be feverish and feel unwell.
- If the mouth is involved there will be pain and difficulty with swallowing.

Signs
- If the maxillary division of the trigeminal nerve is involved, the hard and soft palates are affected, unilaterally.
- If the mandibular division, extensive unilateral cutaneous lesions will be present.

- With ophthalmic division involvement (Gasserian herpes) serious corneal ulceration may develop.
- The unilateral distribution of the lesions along the anatomical distribution of the dermatome is characteristic of herpes zoster.
- Unilateral groups of thin-walled vesicles or ulcers (intraoral) stop sharply at the midline.
- New lesions occur over a period of some 3 weeks.
- There may be pyrexia and regional lymph node enlargement and tenderness.
- The virus is spread by direct contact with vesicular fluid. This will cause chicken pox in those with no previous exposure to herpes zoster. Such spread should be avoided, particularly to pregnant women and the immunosuppressed.
- A painful complication of herpes zoster infection is post-herpetic neuralgia.

Keywords
Unilateral, anatomical, distribution of lesions
Pain precedes vesicle formation

Treatment

- In severe cases and where health is already compromised, aciclovir may be used (800 mg 5 times daily for 5 days).
- Refer for specialist care when the ophthalmic division is involved. Intravenous medication is indicated to avoid loss of sight.

Post-herpetic neuralgia

MH. Previous history of herpes zoster.

- Occurs in up to 10% of patients with herpes zoster affecting the trigeminal nerve.
- The ophthalmic division of the trigeminal nerve is most commonly affected.

Symptoms

- Characterized by persistent (not paroxysmal), unilateral, very severe, dull/boring pain.
- A history of previous skin lesions and any scarring from these aids the diagnosis.

Signs

- Overlying skin is often red as patients may scratch at the skin to gain temporary relief from the pain.

- Pain may be so severe and persistent as to lead to suicidal depression and possible deliberate self-harm.

> *Keywords*
> Continuous, severe, unilateral pain
> Previous herpes zoster infection

Treatment
- Refer for specialist care. No treatment is fully effective. Tricyclic antidepressants, anticonvulsants and local anaesthetic creams may be tried.

Geniculate herpes (Ramsay–Hunt syndrome)

- Caused by herpes zoster infection of the geniculate ganglion.
- Pain occurs in the throat or ear, followed by vesicular eruption on the ear and fauces.
- A lower motor neurone facial palsy (see below) is evident.
- May be accompanied by tinnitus and vertigo.

Treatment
Refer for specialist care.

Bell's palsy

- Acute lower motor neurone (see below) palsy of the facial nerve, usually caused by localized herpes simplex infection, leading to oedema of the nerve in the facial canal.
- Bell's palsy is common, affects both sexes equally, and is usually found in adults.
- In 10% of patients recovery from facial paralysis is incomplete.
- While unilateral facial paralysis is the major presenting problem with Bell's palsy, pain may precede or accompany the palsy.

Symptoms
- Pain around the ear occurs in 50% of patients, prior to or with the onset of paralysis, and may radiate to the jaw.
- Facial paralysis is usually of rapid onset, and at its worst within 48 hours. Paralysis of facial muscles is unilateral.
- Patients may be concerned that they have experienced a stroke (cerebrovascular accident) and need to be reassured that this is not the case.

Signs

- Diagnosis of the cause of pain becomes apparent when paralysis sets in a few hours or days later.
- On testing of the facial muscles, when paralysis has occurred, the patient will be unable to approximate the eye lids or smile on the affected side.

> *Keywords*
> Unilateral pain around ear
> Followed closely by unilateral facial palsy

Treatment

- Refer for specialist care, where prednisolone, perhaps in combination with aciclovir may be used.

Notes:

- The muscles of facial expression are supplied by the seventh cranial (facial) nerve. The neurones which control movement of the muscles of the upper part of the face are innervated from both cerebral hemispheres. In contrast, neurones controlling muscles of the lower face are innervated only from the opposite hemisphere.
- Facial muscle weakness may be caused by primary muscle disease (e.g. myasthenia gravis) or facial nerve lesions.
- Facial nerve lesions may be:
  Upper motor neurone lesion: A lesion above the pontine nucleus causes lower facial paralysis. The upper part of the face is not involved, due to its bilateral innervation.
  Lower motor neurone lesion: The lesion is between the pontine nucleus and the periphery. Both the upper and the lower facial muscles are involved. The commonest cause is Bell's palsy.
- Lower facial muscles are tested by asking the patient to smile or show the teeth.
- Upper facial muscles are tested by asking the patient to 'screw up' the eyes or wrinkle the forehead.

Differential diagnosis of facial palsy

Neurologic:

Bell's palsy
Stroke
Cerebral tumour
Surgery/trauma to facial nerve
Multiple sclerosis

HIV disease
Diabetes mellitus
Ramsay–Hunt syndrome
Guillain–Barré syndrome
Botulism

Primary muscle disease:
Myasthenia gravis

Parotid salivary gland lesions:
Surgery/trauma
Malignancy

Middle ear disorder:
Mastoiditis
Malignancy

Other:
Reiter's syndrome
Melkersson–Rosenthal syndrome

Multiple (disseminated) sclerosis

MH. Possible trigeminal neuralgia.

- Can mimic other causes of dental and non-dental pain, e.g. trigeminal neuralgia.
- Approximately 3% patients presenting with trigeminal neuralgia have multiple sclerosis.
- 50% more women than men are affected.
- The disease is usually first diagnosed at age 20–40 years. It is rarely first diagnosed under 15 and over 50 years.

Symptoms

- Retrobulbar neuritis may cause ocular pain.
- Multiple neurological lesions (e.g. paraesthesia, motor defect, incontinence, visual disturbance) may be present (caused by nerve demyelination). There may be a previous history of such problems disseminated in time and location.
- There will be muscular weakness, tingling or numbness of hands or feet, loss of postural sense, vertigo and sphincter disturbances.
- While remissions are frequent, there can be a progressive deterioration in health.
- Facial pain usually occurs late in the disease, when the diagnosis of multiple sclerosis has usually already been made.

Keywords
Multiple neurological lesions
Disseminated in time and location

Intracranial tumours

Note: All expanding lesions inside the skull, including abscesses, haematomas as well as neoplasms, may give rise to similar symptoms and signs.

- In adults, the commonest intracranial neoplasms are gliomas, meningiomas, metastatic carcinoma (from lung or breast), neuroma (usually eighth nerve) and pituitary tumours.
- In children, the commonest intracranial neoplasms are medulloblastoma and astrocytoma.

Symptoms:

- Recurrent headache, aggravated or precipitated by straining or coughing.
- Vomiting (usually associated with tumours of the posterior fossa and due to direct involvement of the vomiting centre).
- Progressive defects of function, both mental and physical, e.g. deafness, visual deterioration, weakness, personality change, intellectual impairment, epilepsy, disturbance of balance.

Signs

- Papilloedema (bulging of the optic disc), due to obstruction of CSF pathways (therefore most common with posterior fossa tumours).
- Focal neurological signs (may serve to localize the tumour) e.g.:

(i) Acoustic neuroma in the cerebello-pontine angle – is the most common tumour affecting the trigeminal nerve. Leads to:

Sensory loss in the distribution of the trigeminal nerve
Absence of corneal reflex
Unilateral deafness
Weakness of the facial muscles if the facial nerve is involved
Nystagmus towards the affected side
Spastic weakness of the opposite leg
Contralateral extensor (Babinski) plantar response

Pain along the distribution of the trigeminal nerve is unusual but when present is usually persistent. However, occasionally the pain may mimic that of trigeminal neuralgia.

(ii) Parasagittal tumour (meningioma) compressing the olfactory nerve causing anosmia.

(iii) Pituitary adenoma causing bitemporal visual field defects.

Diagnostic tests
Cranial nerve examination (see pages 56–67).
Refer for specialist neurological examination and tests.

Causalgia

- Pain arising after injury to a peripheral sensory nerve, for example, following a difficult extraction.
- Pain is due to aberrant nerve repair.

MH. May follow several weeks after surgery or trauma.

Symptoms
- Constant, burning or boring pain at a site of previous trauma or surgery; can sometimes mimic trigeminal neuralgia.

Signs
- Scarring from previous surgery or trauma.

Keywords
Scarring at site of pain

Diagnostic tests
- Pain can be relieved by administration of a diagnostic local anaesthetic.

Treatment
- Refer for specialist care. No treatment appears to be entirely satisfactory but carbamazepine may be helpful.

2. Vascular origin

Migraine

- Usually starts in the second decade and diminishes with age.
- Women (75%) are more affected than men and the condition may be more common in professional persons.
- One in ten people will have a migraine attack at some time in their life.
- In 50% of cases there is a family history of migraine. Those with a close relative with migraine are likely to have a more severe form of the condition.
- The probable cause is an initial constriction of branches of the

external carotid artery, causing the characteristic aura, followed by dilatation, causing the headache.

Symptoms

- Prodromal (preheadache) stage causes lethargy, an 'aura' (visual disturbance) and tingling of the face and occasionally the mouth. Prodromal stage lasts 15–30 minutes and is followed by severe, throbbing, temporal, frontal and orbital pain.
- Pain is usually unilateral (but sides may change) and of a deep throbbing type. Headache may last 12 hours but usually occurs during the day rather than at night. The frequency of attack is variable.
- The patient is obviously ill, pale, sweating and nauseous. Vomiting may occur.
- Patients prefer to lie in a quiet darkened room (photophobia) and refuse food.
- Attacks occur every few weeks or months.
- An attack may be initiated by psychological stress or some foods, notably red wine, beer, chocolate and cheese. Conversely, starvation may also precipitate an attack.
- Patients may be of an obsessional personality type and attacks may occur during a period of relaxation following intense activity (weekend migraine). Attacks may also may occur premenstrually.
- Indeed, anything that can initiate a headache in a healthy person can initiate migraine in the susceptible.

Keywords
Throbbing day-time headache lasting several hours
Aura
Photophobia
Nausea and vomiting

Treatment

- Simple analgesics and anti-emetics can provide some transient relief. However, it may be best in patients with recurrent bouts to refer. Ergotamine and Sumatriptan may be used.

Periodic migrainous neuralgia (sphenopalatine neuralgia, 'cluster headache', 'alarm clock' headache)

- Caused by arterial spasm and dilatation, like classic migraine.
- May be due to a disorder of the maxillary branch of the external carotid artery (usually) but can involve any vessel, including the internal carotid artery.

- Mainly affects young adults (20–40 years, often students, never under 20 years).
- Males are affected far more often than females (unlike classic migraine).

MH. Often a history of migraine as a child or a family history of migraine. Stress or alcohol may precipitate an attack.

Symptoms
- Unilateral, paroxysmal, dull/boring/burning pain, so severe that the patient cannot function normally.
- Unlike classic migraine, pain usually occurs at night. It is one of the few pain conditions that can awaken a patient from sleep. This observation is useful for diagnosis.
- The pain is episodic (therefore 'periodic' migrainous neuralgia), usually occuring once per 24 hours.
- Pain is of rapid onset and short duration, usually lasting up to 30 minutes only, but occasionally up to 2 hours.
- The pain goes as quickly as it comes.
- Pain is usually limited to the area around and behind the eye and related maxilla.
- Attacks recur at similar times of the night ('alarm clock wakening') and are clustered (often once every 24 hours) and followed by a long period of remission for weeks, months or even years (hence 'cluster headache'). Between bouts there is total relief from pain.
- Autonomic symptoms may accompany periodic migrainous neuralgia including nasal blockage (stuffy nose), nasal discharge and a bloodshot, tearful eye.
- Unlike migraine, there is no nausea or visual disturbance.
- Unlike trigeminal neuralgia, no trigger zone will be found.
- Importantly, for the dentist, 50% of patients with periodic migrainous neuralgia present as toothache.

Keywords
Mainly males
Very severe pain
Episodic (periodic)
Similar time, often at night ('alarm clock awakening')
Occurs in bouts ('cluster headache')
Autonomic symptoms

Treatment
- Refer. Ergotamine or anti-inflammatory drugs, e.g. Indomethacin may be employed. The patient should avoid alcohol.

Differential diagnosis
Sinusitis
Retrobulbar neuritis
Giant cell arteritis
Acute glaucoma
Classic migraine
Trigeminal neuralgia

Paroxysmal facial hemicrania

- Very similar to periodic migrainous neuralgia but without the autonomic problems.

Treatment
- Refer. Indomethacin may be used.

Giant cell (temporal, cranial) arteritis

- Giant cell arteritis is the preferred terminology since the temporal artery is not the only artery that can be involved in this arteritis. Occasionally, similar lesions occur throughout the skeletal muscles, related to their vasculature; this condition has been termed 'polymyalgia arteritica'.
- Pain is caused by ischaemia resulting from the arteritis.
- Giant cell arteritis is uncommon, affects far more females than males and is restricted to the elderly (over 60 years).

Symptoms
- Severe, unilateral ache restricted to the temporal and frontal areas (i.e. side of head and behind the eye).
- The pain is described as dull/boring in character and reaches a crescendo over several days then remains fairly constant.
- Pain can be brought on by eating due to ischaemia of the masticatory muscles (known as masseteric claudication).
- The temporal and frontal skin and scalp may be tender to the touch.
- The patient feels unwell and may suffer aching and stiffness of the shoulders and hips, termed 'polymyalgia rheumatica'.
- This is one of the few pain disorders with systemic upset, e.g. lethargy, weight loss, weakness.
- Nausea may occur and may lead to an erroneous diagnosis of migraine.
- Ocular symptoms include loss of vision in one part of the visual field — this is a *serious* complication.

Signs
- The temporal arteries may be occluded, pulseless, thickened and tortuous.

Keywords
Elderly, females
Unilateral, boring pain
Masseteric claudication
Systemic upset

Diagnostic tests
- Multiple temporal artery biopsies are needed as giant cell lesions occur sporadically along the nerve ('skip' lesions)
- The ESR (or plasma viscosity, or C-reactive protein) is notably elevated.

Treatment
- Hospital must be alerted immediately since a rapid deterioration in vision will occur if the retinal arteries are involved (25+% of patients).
- Acute necrosis of facial tissues may occur (rarely) such as gangrene of the scalp, lip or tongue.
- Specialist treatment may include using high-dose corticosteroids.

Cardiac ischaemia

MH. Pre-existing heart or circulatory disease, hypertension, diabetes mellitus.

Symptoms
- Pain may refer to the left arm and left jaw, and may be related to exercise, eating a large meal and emotion.
- Pain lasts a few minutes only and is relieved by rest.
- Attacks occur most often in cold weather.

Signs
- Diagnosis is by history.

Treatment
- Refer for medical assessment and treatment.

3. Maxillary antrum/nasopharynx

Sinusitis

- Infection (usually bacterial) of the maxillary sinus.

MH. History of recent cold or recurrent sinusitis.

DH. Possible history of a recent tooth extraction, causing an oro-antral fistula. Periapical infection of an upper posterior tooth.

Symptoms

- Usually unilateral, rarely bilateral, dull/throbbing, continuous pain, limited to the upper jaw and under the eye.
- Pain is worse in the evening and with bending or shaking of the head and lying down.
- Patients may experience the feeling of fluid moving in the affected sinus.
- The associated stuffy nose, nasal discharge and fullness of cheek may be described as a 'cold in the head'.
- Pressure over the cheek causes pain and many upper teeth, on one side, may be painful.
- The patient may feel feverish and unwell.

Signs

- In an otherwise healthy patient, there is never any facial swelling associated with sinusitis. However, facial swelling may occasionally be seen with severe sinus infections in patients with diabetes mellitus or the immunocompromised.
- There will be signs of nasal obstruction with mucopurulent rhinorrhoea.
- A number of maxillary teeth (usually molars) may be periostitic, equally tender to percussion yet vital (differentiates from periapical periodontitis, which usually affects a single non-vital tooth), otherwise there will be an absence of dental signs.

Keywords
Unilateral pain under eye
Numerous maxillary teeth on one side may be painful
Stuffy nose
Fluid level (see below)

Diagnostic tests

- Transillumination of the antra or an occipitomental radiograph may show a fluid level or thickening of the antral lining.

Treatment

- Antibiotics, e.g. erythromycin, trimethoprin, amoxycillin or ampicillin 250 mg, four times per day for five days, plus a nasal decongestant (0.1% xylometazoline HCl) and inhalants.

- Refer if persistent. Antral washout or surgery may be recommended in severe/recurrent disease.

Malignancy (see also Chapters 10 and 12):

- Any tumour arising along the intra- or extracranial course of the trigeminal nerve or within the nasopharynx or maxillary antrum may cause unilateral, dull, facial pain.
- The most common malignancy affecting the maxillary antrum is squamous cell carcinoma.
- The prognosis is poor since diagnosis is usually late. The onset is insidious and symptoms are initially absent or trivial (often mimicking chronic sinusitis).
- A tumour may spread from the antrum in any direction:

The anterior and infratemporal walls of the antrum are thin and tumours can readily erode them to appear as a swelling on the cheek, mimicking a dental abscess.

A tumour may penetrate the floor of the antrum to present as a swelling on the palate or buccal sulcus, mimicking a dental abscess. If a maxillary denture is used, it may no longer fit. The tumour may appear as a fungating mass or an ulcer with raised, rolled and everted edges. Occasionally, a tumour may extrude through a recent extraction socket, mimicking an antral prolapse. Teeth may be loosened and painful as a result of bone destruction, mimicking periodontal disease. The dental pulp may necrose as a result of disruption of the blood supply. Thus, an acute dental abscess may be the first presenting sign of the malignancy.

A tumour eroding the posterior wall may damage the posterior superior alveolar nerves, resulting in anaesthesia of the teeth and gum in the maxillary molar region. Extension into the infratemporal fossa may involve the sphenopalatine ganglion and result in anaesthesia or paraesthesia of the palate. Alternatively, the maxillary nerve may be damaged leading to anaesthesia of the upper face and lip. If the medial pterygoid muscle is involved, trismus may result.

The roof of the antrum is very thin and easily eroded. Extension here may involve the infra-orbital nerve resulting in facial anaesthesia, alteration of the pupillary level (as the eye is pushed up), proptosis (drooping of the eyelid) and diplopia (double vision). Tears may spill onto the face (epiphora) due to blockage of the nasolacrimal duct.

A tumour may extend into the nasal cavity causing partial obstruction and nasal discharge.

Symptoms and signs

- Occur late in the disease process.
- Depend upon the direction of spread (see above).
- May mimic those of other dental and non-dental diseases.

Diagnostic tests

- Lymph node examination (see also pages 14 and 17). Drainage from the maxillary antrum is to the submandibular and upper deep cervical nodes. Lymphadenopathy may indicate metastatic spread. However, the intermediary retropharyngeal nodes cannot be palpated and metastasis may thus be missed.
- Transillumination – early lesions will not be visible.
- Refer for specialist examination and tests. These may include sinuscopy, radiography (occipitomental views will not show early erosions), tomography and biopsy.

Trotter's syndrome

- Nasopharyngeal tumour causing pain in the lower jaw, tongue and side of head, and middle ear deafness.
- May occur in 30% nasopharyngeal tumours.
- Any pain remaining undiagnosed must be referred to exclude serious underlying pathology.
- Acoustic neuroma (tumour of eighth cranial nerve) is notorious for mimicking other causes of facial pain.
- Unfortunately, in terms of detection, pain is rarely a symptom of early oral cancer.

4. Salivary glands (see Chapters 8, 12 and 13)

5. Oral mucosa: Zoster and geniculate herpes (see pages 103–105)

6. Jaws/masticatory muscles

Temporomandibular joint disorders include:

Temporomandibular joint pain-dysfunction syndrome
Osteoarthritis
Rheumatoid arthritis
Trauma
Developmental defects
Ankylosis

Infection
Neoplasia

Temporomandibular joint pain-dysfunction syndrome (PDS) (facial arthromyalgia)

- This is the most common problem in or around the temporomandibular joints.
- Equal frequency between genders but five times as many females seek treatment. Usually affects patients aged between 15 and 40 years.

Symptoms

- Unilateral or bilateral, dull pain within the temporomandibular joint (TMJ) and/or surrounding muscles, sometimes on waking or during eating or speech.
- If bilateral, one side is usually most affected.
- Occasionally, the TMJ may lock open or closed.
- TMJ sounds, such as clicking, crunching or grating are often described.
- Headaches, facial pain and neck related aches are reported.
- Any headache is usually located in the temporal region, often on waking, but may extend into the day. The pain is usually a dull ache. Unlike migraine, there are no associated features, such as photophobia or nausea.
- Pain is cyclical and usually resolves, but may recur.
- On questioning, some patients reveal that the problem started, or is exacerbated, by psychological stress.

Signs

- Joint clicks may occur. The click may be caused by noise generated by displacement of the articular disc from the head of the condyle and then escaping into the correct position. However, joint clicks are common in patients without PDS.
- Pain may be elicited on palpation of the TMJ and masticatory muscles (see Chapter 3). The masticatory muscles may be hypertrophic (due to parafunction such as nocturnal bruxism).
- Mandibular movement may be limited and deviation may occur on the opening or closing cycle.
- Oral habits, such as parafunction, can be identified in 50% of subjects.
- Bruxism is suggested by observation of scalloping of the lateral borders of the tongue, ridging of the buccal mucosa, tooth wear, faceting, restoration wear, fracture, dentine exposure and sensitivity.

- Occlusal disharmony is no longer considered to be a primary aetiological factor in PDS. However, it is possible that occlusal interferences may be contributing factors in the aetiology of bruxism.

Psychological considerations

- Only a small minority of patients experiencing PDS have a mental disorder but any chronic pain may affect patients psychologically.
- Anxiety, depression and somatoform disorders (including hypochondria) are contributory (and often accompanying) factors to PDS.
- The prevalence of depression in PDS is five times greater than in the general population.

Diagnostic tests

- Clinical and radiographic examination usually reveals no joint pathology.
- As radiographic joint changes only arise with degenerative disease, diagnosis of PDS is by exclusion of organic disease.
- Isolated headache or painless joint sounds are *not* diagnostic of PDS.

Keywords
More females present
Unilateral or bilateral dull ache, related to TMJ and/or surrounding muscles
Bruxism
Psychological stress
No TMJ pathology

Treatment

- Since in most instances symptoms are self-limiting, treatment should be conservative and reversible.
- Provide information about the problem, emphasizing its frequency and self-limiting nature.
- Soft diet, elimination of chewing gum.
- Application of moist heat or ultrasound to painful muscles and physiotherapy have been suggested to be of benefit.
- Analgesics.
- Anxiolytics (e.g. diazepam (muscle relaxant and anxiolytic) 5 mg 1 hour before sleep, then 2 mg twice daily, for up to 10 days maximum).
- Antidepressants.

- Occlusal splints (various).
- Occlusal adjustment of the natural teeth by selective grinding is irreversible and *not* recommended.

Osteoarthritis
- Rare.
- Crepitation (crunching and grating) is the joint sound; crepitus denotes degenerative joint disease.
- May be accompanied by preauricular pain, but not involving the masticatory muscles.
- Radiographs (e.g. panoramic, transpharyngeal, transcranial oblique lateral, open and closed) will show degenerative joint disease.

Rheumatoid arthritis
- Crepitation is the joint sound.
- The TMJ is rarely symptomatic and diagnosis of the disease in other joints has usually already been made.

Trauma
- Condyle fracture or traumatic arthritis. Pain and trismus of traumatic arthritis resolve after one week. Microtrauma from parafunction may result in chronic symptoms.
- Dislocation is usually a result of trauma, and is rare. Very rarely, dislocation occurs after yawning.

Developmental defects
- Rare.
- Includes hyperplasia (most common — leads to increasing facial and occlusal deformity), hypoplasia, aplasia.

Ankylosis (rare in developed countries)
- Following trauma, infection or other inflammatory condition.

Infection (rare in developed countries)
- Following penetrating trauma to the joint or spreading from middle ear or other structures.

Neoplasia (rare)
- Osteoma, chondroma, chondrosarcoma, secondary carcinoma.

7. Ears

Otitis media (inflammation of the middle ear)

- May present to the dentist as pain in the region of the temporomandibular joint.

- Rarely, infection may spread to cause an infective arthritis of the temporomandibular joint.
- May involve the facial (seventh cranial) nerve leading to unilateral facial paralysis.
- Some 50% of cerebral abscesses result from extension of infection from the middle ear.

8. Eyes

Glaucoma

- Due to rapid increase in intraocular pressure.

Symptoms
- Persistent, severe, unilateral orbital pain, centred above the eye but may radiate across one side of the face.
- Vomiting and loss of vision may occur.

Signs
- The eye is stony hard, due to raised intraocular pressure.
- The pupil is dull, sea green, oval and dilated. The cornea is misty.

Treatment
- Immediate referral to ophthalmology.

9. Psychogenic

Atypical facial pain

- A significant proportion of patients presenting with facial pain will be suffering from atypical facial pain.
- However, the diagnosis cannot be made until all other possibilities are excluded.
- Since no organic lesion can be found in atypical facial pain, it is tempting to dismiss the pain as 'all in the mind'. However, the pain associated with psychogenic pain is no more or less real than inflammation of the pulp to the patient experiencing it. If untreated, some patients may attempt suicide.
- It should also be remembered that psychogenic pain does not confer immunity to caries or carcinoma.

MH. Possible history of depression or anxiety.

DH. Patient may have attended many dentists, doctors and other specialists in failed attempts to cure the pain. Patients may have experienced serial extraction of teeth in an attempt to eliminate the pain.

- Mainly females (70%) are affected, usually adults.

Symptoms
- The pain is described as a vague, constant, dull ache, present all day every day. It is poorly localized, although the maxilla is often involved.
- The pain may start unilaterally but often spreads to cross the midline (unlike other facial pains).
- The continuous nature of the pain, often for years, the lack of provoking and relieving factors and the inconsistency with clinical findings (no pathology identified) are characteristic.
- Despite the pain being described as unbearable, sleep is not affected.
- The pain is not consistent with anatomical boundaries or distribution of nerves. Thus, pain may be described as crossing over the midline of the face, or be bilateral, or involve two or more sensory nerve fields.
- The description of the pain is occasionally bizarre, such as 'like ants crawling over my face'.
- Patients may present with a detailed written list of problems and dates.

Signs
- No causative factor is detectable.
- Cranial nerves are intact.
- Often, there will be variable or inconsistent responses to vitality tests.

Keywords
Mainly adult females
Continuous (for months or years), unchanging pain
Non-anatomical distribution
Bizarre description
No signs
Sleep not affected

Treatment
- Refer to an appropriate clinic (e.g. pain clinic, liaison psychiatry). Patients should be offered the opportunity to be examined by a psychiatrist, as therapy is typically psychiatric in nature (e.g. psychotherapy, anxiolytics, anti-depressants). Furthermore, a depressed patient in continuous pain may attempt suicide.

Atypical odontalgia

Atypical facial pain where the patient attributes the pain to the teeth.

Symptoms

- The aetiology and symptomatology are the same as those of atypical facial pain but the patient more definitely associates the pain with the teeth.
- Many dental treatments may have been attempted, by different dentists, including serial extraction, with no improvement in the pain.
- Following extirpation of a pulp, or extraction of a suspected tooth, the pain migrates elsewhere but usually near by (i.e. to the next tooth).

Signs

- None; diagnosis is by exclusion.

Treatment

- Stop dental treatment and refer to an appropriate clinic (see above).

Burning mouth syndrome (burning tongue, glossopyrosis, glossodynia, stomatodynia)

- The vast majority of patients are female (F:M 7:1), aged 50 years or more.
- The aetiology includes psychological factors such as anxiety, cancerophobia, hypochondria and depression.

Symptoms

- Severe, constant, burning pain, often bilateral and present for months or years.
- Pain is often relieved by eating.
- The tongue is involved most often but any mucous membranes may be affected.
- Despite the constancy and severity of the pain, sleep is not affected.

Signs

- No mucous membrane abnormalities can be seen in the area affected.

Diagnostic tests (to exclude organic disease) may include:
- Haematology.
- Thyroid function.
- Examine dentures.
- Salivary flow test.
- Examine for parafunction.
- Swab/smear/oral rinse to test for candidal infection (see page 159).

For psychological factors:
- Cancerophobia — Ask the patient to rate their fear of cancer on a scale of 0 to 10, where 0 indicates no fear at all and 10 indicates an overwhelming concern.
- Regular self-examination of the mouth by observation in a mirror may suggest cancerophobia.
- Patients may have a friend of relative who has been diagnosed with cancer.

Treatment
- When other factors have been excluded, the patient should be referred for detailed psychiatric assessment.
- Antidepressants and cognitive behavioural therapy may be helpful.

Differential diagnosis of burning mouth

Psychogenic
- Burning mouth syndrome

Deficiency states
- Vitamin B
- Iron
- Folic acid

Infections
- Candidiasis

Other
- Denture discomfort
- Dry mouth
- Allergy
- Diabetes mellitus

Further reading

Gray, R.J.M., Davies, S.J. and Quayle, A.A. (1995) *Temporomandibular Disorders: A Clinical Approach*. London: British Dental Association.

Scully, C., Flint, S.R. and Porter, S.R. (1996) *Oral Diseases: An illustrated guide to diagnosis and management of diseases of the oral mucosa, gingivae, teeth, salivary glands, bones and joints*, 2nd edn. London: Martin Dunitz.

7

Trauma

Summary

Introduction

Traumatic injuries of:
1. Teeth, periodontal ligament and alveolar bone
2. Mandible (fracture and dislocation)
3. Maxilla (Le Fort I, II and III)
4. Malar complex
5. Soft tissue injuries
6. Tooth surface loss/tooth wear (abrasion, attrition, erosion and abfraction)

Iatrogenic trauma (resulting from treatment, e.g. oro-antral fistula, mandibular fracture, mandibular dislocation)

Introduction

It is essential to take a detailed history (see Chapter 2) for all traumatic injuries to the face, teeth and oral mucosa. A dental practitioner may be required to provide a report for a court, solicitors or for insurance purposes. Drawings and clinical photographs will support a detailed history and clinical examination.

However, the history will have to be postponed when the following essential first aid measures are required:

Airway – Establish and maintain the airway, e.g. remove foreign bodies from the oral cavity, insert airway.
Bleeding – Arrest haemorrhage.
Consciousness – Assess level of consciousness of patient.

N.B.
- In *all* cases of trauma, where there may be serious bodily injury, call an ambulance to transport the patient to the nearest Accident and Emergency Department.

- Always refer patients for medical examination when any non-dental injury is suspected.

History

The following questions should be asked of the patient or an accompanying adult if the patient is too young or distressed:

- When did the injury happen?
  The prognosis for avulsed teeth is significantly affected by the time the tooth is out of the mouth and how it is stored during this time (see page 129).
- How did the injury happen?
  e.g. Assault, road traffic accidents, sports and industrial injuries where there may be future litigation.
- Did you lose consciousness?
  If yes, the patient must be referred to a hospital for neurological assessment and further investigations, e.g. skull X-rays and observation overnight.
- Have the police been informed (or will they be)?
  (Possible future litigation.)
- Is your bite altered?
  e.g. Fractured mandible/maxilla, displaced teeth, dislocation of mandible.
- Can you open your mouth fully?
  e.g. Trismus with fractured mandible/condyles/zygomatic arch.
- Can you close your mouth?
  Anterior open bite occurs with bilateral condylar fractures and Le Fort fractures. All teeth apart indicates dislocation.
- Do you have any numbness?
  Lower lip with mandibular fracture, due to trauma to the inferior alveolar nerve. Cheek with zygomatic fracture due to trauma to the infra-orbital nerve.
- Do you have double vision?
  Fractured malar/maxilla/orbital floor.
- Are any teeth missing?
  All teeth must be accounted for. Check with radiographs for foreign bodies in lips and face, lungs and gastrointestinal tract.

1. Teeth, periodontal ligament and alveolar bone

For examination see also Chapter 3.

Enamel-only fractures

Symptoms
- May be asymptomatic.
- Sharp tooth, lacerating the soft tissues of the mouth.
- Pain on biting.

Signs
- Loss of enamel.
- Hairline cracks in the enamel.

Diagnostic tests

Radiology
- Periapical views (to rule out root fractures or tooth displacement)
- Soft tissue views, e.g. lips, are required when there is missing tooth structure which cannot be accounted for.

Transillumination:
- Ideally with magnification, will show up enamel cracks.

N.B. Cracked cusps see pages 78–80.

Enamel and dentine

Symptoms
- Sharp tooth.
- Sensitivity to temperature change.
- Pain on biting.

Diagnostic tests
As for enamel fractures.

N.B. Vitality testing at this time may be unreliable due to concussion to the pulp.

Treatment options
- Smooth sharp teeth.
- Restore with composite or etch and rebond the broken

fragment. The latter is the treatment of choice when the fragment is available.

Important notes: Traumatized teeth must be monitored regularly to ensure that vitality is not lost. All involved teeth, including those that are symptom free, should be tested 6 weeks to 2 months after the initial injury, with thermal and electric pulp tests. Repeat X-rays at 3 months are also required to ensure that there are no apical changes. Loss of vitality can also present as discoloration of a tooth due to pulpal haemorrhage into the dentinal tubules or as pain in a previously asymptomatic tooth.

Fractures involving the pulp

Symptoms
- Pain and sensitivity. Often severe to temperature change or biting.

Signs
- Often extensive tooth loss and visible pulpal exposure.

Diagnostic tests
Radiology
- Periapical views.
- Occlusal views are useful for examining several adjacent traumatized teeth in the anterior region.

Treatment options include:
- Dressing pinpoint exposures with calcium hydroxide and restoring with composite or rebond the fragment.
- Pulpotomy in teeth with open apices.
- Pulpectomy and root canal therapy.
- Extraction of teeth which are unrestorable.

Root fractures

These may be in the apical third, middle or coronal third of a tooth.

Symptoms
- Pain and often loosening of teeth.

Signs
- Pain on palpation and increased mobility.

Diagnostic tests

- Periapical radiographs confirm the diagnosis. The film should always be viewed dry (following processing) in order to diagnose root fractures accurately.

Treatment options

- Rigid splinting of teeth for 2–3 months with apical third fractures.
- Middle third fractures – splinting of teeth for 2–3 months, though the prognosis is much less favourable.
- Coronal third – extraction or orthodontic extrusion of the root may be necessary. The prognosis is very poor when the fracture is close to the gingival crevice.
- As above, teeth must also be monitored for loss of vitality, in which case root canal therapy is necessary.
- In addition to crown and root fractures, teeth may also be displaced when there is damage to the periodontal ligament and surrounding alveolar bone.

Definitions

Concussion

- Trauma to the pulp and periodontal ligament. The tooth is not obviously displaced or loose.

Subluxation

- The tooth is loosened but not displaced. There is no apparent injury to the alveolar bone of the socket.

Displacement

- The tooth is displaced together with damage to the alveolar bone.

Avulsion

- Tooth completely out of the socket.

Symptoms

- Pain.
- Loose tooth/teeth.
- Missing tooth/teeth.
- Altered bite with subluxation and displacement.

Diagnostic tests

Radiology

- Intra-oral periapical and occlusal views.

N.B. When treating avulsed teeth:

- Ideally the tooth should be rinsed in water and immediately replaced in its socket. If not possible, it should be stored in milk or placed in the patient's buccal sulcus provided their level of consciousness permits and they are old enough not to swallow it!
- Reposition and splint for 10 days.
- Root canal therapy is required for avulsed teeth with closed apices after 10 days.
- Subluxation and displacement injuries will also frequently require root canal therapy.
- Long-term follow-up is required to check for root resorption, ankylosis or obliteration of the root canal by secondary dentine.
- Antibiotics are recommended for avulsion and subluxation injuries and also for soft tissue trauma.
- The tetanus status of the patient should also be assessed and a booster dose of toxoid administered when necessary.

Deciduous teeth

- Avulsed deciduous teeth should not be reimplanted as they may become infected and damage the permanent successor or loosen and be inhaled. Space maintenance using orthodontic brackets and wires may be required, depending on the age of the child and the tooth involved.
- Deciduous teeth that are very mobile should be removed.
- Intruded teeth may also cause damage to the permanent successor.
- They can either be extracted or left to erupt.

2. Mandible (fracture and dislocation)

Mandibular fractures (Fig. 7.1)

Aetiology

- Trauma
- Pathological fracture due to cystic expansion, (see Chapter 9), neoplasms (primary or secondary) and infection, e.g. osteomyelitis, which weaken the mandible so that minimal trauma, e.g. eating, will result in a fracture of the jaw.

Symptoms

- Pain.

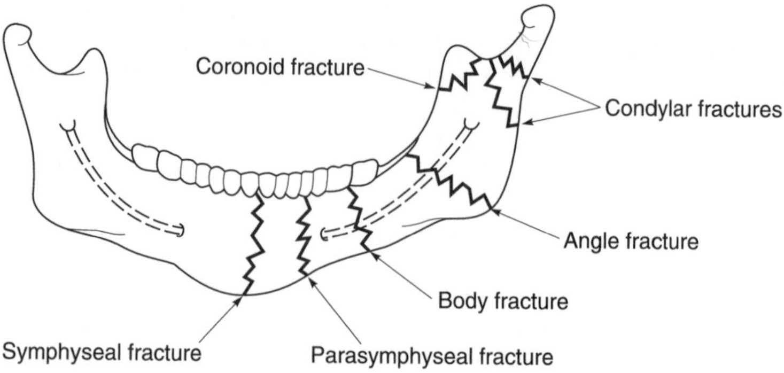

Figure 7.1 Mandibular fracture sites.

- Limitation of movement.
- Bleeding either intra-orally or from the ear (in cases of condylar fracture, as a result of laceration of the skin of the external auditory meatus).
- Altered bite.
- Numbness of the lower lip due to trauma of the inferior alveolar nerve.
- Swelling.

Signs
- Facial oedema and ecchymosis (bruising).
- Trismus and limitation of movement.
- Deformity of the contour of the mandible.
- Palpable step deformity. (Palpation of the posterior and lower borders of the mandible will identify a step in the normally smooth bony contour of the jaw.)
- Abnormal mobility of the bone and crepitus.

- **Crepitus** is a grating sound heard on movement of the bone at the fracture site. To test for crepitus, place the forefingers of both hands on the teeth or bone on either side of the fracture and the thumbs on the lower border of the mandible. *Gentle* movement of the bone ends will cause the sound to be heard.

- Tenderness on palpation.
- Occlusal derangement.
- Intra-orally, there may be bleeding and/or ecchymosis.
- Abnormal mobility of teeth adjacent to the fracture.
- In order to elicit all the signs, examinations must be comprehensive and methodical (see also Chapter 3).

- Extra-oral examination should start at the condyles noting any tenderness on palpation. *Note:* Compare both sides. A fractured condyle will not move when the patient opens his/her mouth. Then palpate the posterior border of the ascending ramus and along the lower border of the mandible to the midline to check for abnormal mobility of the jaw, crepitus and step deformities.
- Intra-oral examination must elicit any swelling, ecchymosis as noted above and abnormal mobility of bone. The occlusion should be examined for any derangement, including anterior open bite, and the teeth need to be examined for mobility, fracture and alveolar fracture (where several teeth move simultaneously).

N.B. Patients sustaining mandibular trauma, particularly a direct blow to the chin, may have multiple cracked teeth (see Chapter 5, pages 78–80).

- A direct blow to the chin may also result in bilateral condylar and midline (symphyseal) fractures. This, the 'guardsman's' fracture, is also seen in soldiers who faint on parade while standing to attention.

Diagnostic tests

Radiology
- Two views taken at 90 degrees to each other will enable an assessment of the displacement of the fracture to be made.

Extra-oral
- Panoral radiograph or right and left lateral oblique views, for body and condylar fractures.
- Postero-anterior view to assess the degree of displacement of fractures of the body of the mandible.
- Reverse Towne's view for condylar fractures.

Intra-oral
- Periapicals and lower occlusal to assess damage to the teeth and alveolar bone. The lower occlusal view is also of particular help in assessing displacement in midline fractures of the mandible.

Dislocation

- Definition: displacement of the condyles from their normal positions within the glenoid fossae. The condyles become fixed anterior to the articular eminences and maintained in this position by muscle spasm.

Aetiology

- Trauma (may be iatrogenic following tooth extraction, especially under sedation or general anaesthesia).
- Yawning or opening mouth widely.
- Occasionally seen in patients on drugs with extrapyramidal effects, e.g. phenothiazines.
- Spontaneous in patients with a history of chronic recurrent dislocation due to laxity of the capsular ligaments and with a flat articular eminence.

Symptoms

- Pain.
- Inability to close mouth.

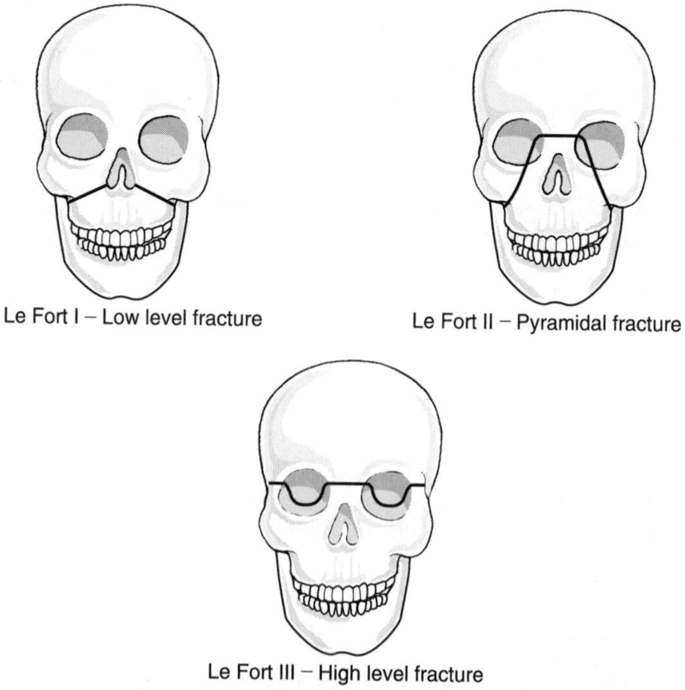

Figure 7.2 Le Fort type classification for fractures of the middle third of the facial skeleton.

Signs
- Mouth wide open and fixed in this position.
- Pain on palpation of the muscles of mastication and condyles.
- Condyles palpable anterior to the articular eminence.
- Dribbling and pooling of saliva due to difficulty swallowing.

Diagnostic tests

Radiology
- Panoral or lateral oblique views confirm condyles anterior to the articular eminences.

Treatment
- Reduction of a dislocated mandible can be achieved by standing behind the patient, placing the thumbs on the posterior mandibular teeth and pressing downwards and backwards to free the condyles before rotating the anterior portion of the mandible upwards. The thumbs should be covered with gauze for protection, since they are likely to be bitten! In cases where there is severe spasm, local anaesthesia, sedation or general anaesthesia may have to be used to effect a reduction. Following reduction, patients must be advised not to open their mouths widely and to support their jaw with their hand to limit opening if they have to yawn.

3. Maxilla (middle third of the face) Le Fort I, II and III

Classification (see Fig. 7.2)
Le Fort I, (Guérin's fracture): a low-level fracture extending across the maxilla between the floor of the maxillary sinus and the floor of the orbit.

Le Fort II: a pyramidal fracture involving the mid-third of the face.

Le Fort III: A high-level fracture resulting in the separation of the facial bones from the neurocranium usually occurs with Le Fort I and Le Fort II fractures.

Symptoms
- Pain.
- Facial swelling.
- Altered bite.
- Double vision, due to entrapment of eye muscles.
- Numbness of the cheek and upper lip, due to trauma to the infra-orbital nerve.

Signs

- Oedema and ecchymosis.
- Bilateral circumorbital ecchymosis.
- Subconjunctival haemorrhage.
- Lengthening of the face.
- Dish-faced deformity due to posterior displacement of the maxilla.
- Malocclusion with anterior open bite.
- Anaesthesia in the distribution of the infra-orbital nerves.
- Diplopia (double vision) on upward gaze.
- The interpupillary line (an imaginary line drawn between the pupils) is angled and no longer horizontal due to fracture of the floor of the orbit.
- Damage to the nose and the medial canthal ligaments results in a traumatic telecanthus (eyes are wider apart).
- Blood and cerebrospinal fluid (a clear, watery fluid) discharging from the nose (CSF rhinorrhoea).

Diagnostic tests

Radiology (refer for)

- Occipito-mental views (10 degrees and 30 degrees).
- Submento-vertex view.
- Lateral skull.
- Postero-anterior jaw view.
- Nasal bone views.

Examination of middle third (maxillary) fractures

- Palpate infra-orbital margins and fronto-zygomatic sutures for step deformities.
- Place the finger of one hand in the palate and the thumb and forefinger of the other hand below the nares on the upper lip, to check for mobility in Le Fort I fractures.
- Place a finger in palate and thumb and forefinger of the other hand over the bridge of the nose and the infra-orbital margins to check for movement in Le Fort II fractures.
- Place a finger and thumb on the fronto-nasal suture and grasp the maxilla. Movement of the entire face is felt in Le Fort III fractures.

4. Malar (zygomatico-maxillary) complex (Fig. 7.3)

Aetiology

As cheek bones are prominent on the facial skeleton, they are frequently fractured by blows to the face, e.g. fights, road traffic accidents and sports injuries.

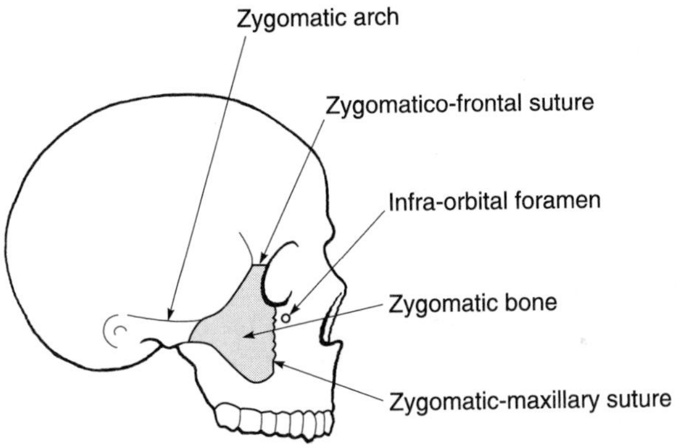

Figure 7.3 Malar (zygomatic) fractures.

Fractures may involve the arch only or the whole of the zygomatic complex including the orbital floor.

An orbital floor fracture with no other injuries to the malar complex is termed an orbital 'blow out' fracture.

Symptoms

- Pain.
- Swelling and ecchymosis.
- Flattened cheek bone.
- Trismus due to the fractured arch impinging on the coronoid process.
- Double vision.
- Numbness of the cheek and upper lip in the region of the distribution of the infra-orbital and anterior superior alveolar nerves.

Signs

- A displaced cheek bone is often best viewed by standing behind the patient and looking down to compare the unaffected and traumatized sides.
- Subconjunctival haemorrhage with no posterior border, i.e. when the patient looks medially the conjunctiva is red due to haemorrhage, from the lateral part of the iris to the outer corner (canthus) of the eye. The blood remains bright red as oxygen can diffuse through the cornea.
- Periorbital ecchymosis (bruising around the eye).
- Step deformities can be felt by palpating the infra-orbital

margin and the frontozygomatic sutures and by comparing both sides. In patients with extensive periorbital oedema and ecchymosis, this may be difficult. However, by keeping gentle finger pressure over the infra-orbital margin, the fluid will be displaced, enabling any step defects to be felt.
- Altered sensation in the distribution of the sensory nerves can be demonstrated by gently touching the skin with a fine probe.
- There may be bleeding from the nose (epistaxis) on the traumatized side.
- The full range of eye movements must be tested to ensure that there is no entrapment of the inferior rectus (limitation of upward gaze) and other eye muscles (see also Chapter 4, page 61).
- Check that the interpupillary line is horizontal.
- It is essential in all fractures of the maxillary and malar complex that visual acuity is monitored pre- and postoperatively, by ophthalmologists, as bleeding into the orbit may cause retinal artery spasm which, if untreated, can result in blindness.

N.B.
- All cases of trauma where fracture of the mandible, maxilla or malar bones is suspected, must be referred to a maxillofacial unit for further assessment and treatment.

Diagnostic tests
Radiology (refer for)
- Occipito-mental views (10 degrees and 30 degrees.)
- Submento-vertex views which demonstrate fractures of the zygomatic arch.
- Tomograms of the orbit for demonstrating 'blow out' fractures.

5. Soft tissue injuries

- Injuries to the oral mucosa and skin frequently occur in conjunction with dental and bony injuries. They may also be the only injuries sustained by the patient.

Symptoms
- Pain, bleeding and swelling at the injury site.
- Careful examination is required to identify sites of haemorrhage. All wounds must be thoroughly debrided and copiously irrigated to remove foreign matter. Tissue that has been

devitalized will need to be removed. Contaminated soft tissue injuries, including animal bites, will require antibiotic prophylaxis and also the tetanus status of the patient must be established. A course of immunization or a booster dose may be required after ensuring the patient has no history of allergy to tetanus toxoid.
- Palpate for solid masses, e.g. in the lip, especially if a tooth or part of a tooth is missing and cannot be accounted for.

Diagnostic tests
- Soft tissue radiographs and chest X-rays will be required when teeth or parts of teeth are missing.

6. Tooth surface loss/tooth wear

- May be multifactorial in aetiology and a combination of the following three causes:

i. Abrasion: is the pathological loss, by wear, of tooth substance or a restoration by factors other than tooth contact. Caused by friction produced when tooth tissue is persistently rubbed.

Aetiology
- Traumatic tooth brushing.
- Wear from rubbing of teeth by pipes and musical instruments.

Symptoms
- May be symptom free or patients may complain of thermal sensitivity due to dentine exposure or acute chronic pulpitis (see pages 76, 80–84).

Signs
- Buccal gingival recession and exposure of root dentine and cementum.

ii. Attrition: is the loss of tooth substance or restoration caused by mastication or tooth-to-tooth contact of occlusal and interproximal surfaces.

Aetiology
- Coarse diet.
- Bruxism or other parafunctional habits.
- Excessive wear due to porcelain or composite restorations in the opposing teeth (differential wear).

Symptoms

- As above – symptom free or sensitivity with extremes of temperature (dentine exposure, acute chronic pulpitis see pages 76, 80–84). In severe cases may lead to acute apical periodontitis and pulp necrosis (see Chapter 5).

Signs

- Tooth surface loss on the occlusal and incisal surfaces, flattening of cusps, worn incisal edges and flattening of contact points between teeth.

iii. Erosion: is the loss of tooth substance by a chemical process not involving bacterial action. Acidic damage is the most common cause, leading to loss of the inorganic matrix.

Aetiology

- Dietary, e.g. acidic and carbonated soft drinks. High consumption of fruit juices (citric acid is a particular problem).
- Gastric reflux, e.g. hiatus hernia and bulimia.

Symptoms

- As above: sensitivity with temperature extremes.
- May ultimately result in pulp necrosis.

Signs

- Tooth surface loss on the occlusal surfaces of the posterior teeth and palatal/lingual surfaces of the anterior teeth.
- Any exposed dentine is smooth and shiny.
- Restorations unaffected by erosion, e.g. amalgam and composite are proud of the adjacent tissue.

iv. Abfraction: is the loss of tooth substance at the cervical region not due to any of the above causes. Symptoms and signs as for abrasion but without evidence or history of traumatic tooth brushing.

Aetiology

- Occlusal forces.
- Excessive tensile and compressive forces cause flexure at the necks of teeth.
- Enamel cracks occur with the eventual loss of tooth substance.
- Patients usually bruxists or elderly.

Iatrogenic trauma

Traumatic injuries may arise due to complications of dental surgery. These include:

- Fracture of the mandible which may occur as a result of excessive force being applied and insufficient bone removal/tooth sectioning during the extraction of an impacted third molar tooth.
- Tuberosity fracture and the creation of an oro-antral fistula when removing an upper molar tooth resulting in a communication between the oral cavity and the maxillary antrum.

Symptoms of an oro-antral communication
- Pain.
- Air entering the mouth when breathing through the nose.
- Fluids taken orally entering the nose through the communication.

Signs
- A smooth, soft tissue swelling (the antral lining) may be visible in the socket. This can be pushed upwards into the antrum.
- Bubbles of air are seen at the extraction site when the patient breathes out.

Diagnostic tests
- Occipito-mental radiographs may show either a fluid level in the maxillary sinus due to bleeding into the antrum and sinusitis, or an opacity due to mucosal infection.
- When the patient tries to breathe out through the nose while pinching the nares, air escapes through the fistula into the oral cavity. Bubbles are seen at the site of the fistula.

Further reading

Andreasen, J.O. and Andreasen, F.M. (1994) *Textbook and Color Atlas of Traumatic Injuries to the Teeth*, 3rd edn. Copenhagen: Munksgaard.

Dimitroulis, C. and Avery, B.S. (1994) *Maxillofacial Injuries – A Synopsis of Basic Principles, Diagnosis and Management*. Oxford: Wright.

8

Infection

Summary

Introduction

1. Bacterial

Dental caries
Osteomyelitis (acute and chronic)
Ludwig's angina
Tuberculosis (see Chapter 10)
Syphilis (see Chapter 10)
Diphtheria
Actinomycosis
Gram negative infections in the immunosupressed patient
Periodontal disease (see Chapter 5)
Acute and chronic apical periodontitis (see Chapter 5)
Acute necrotizing ulcerative gingivitis (see Chapter 5)
Lateral periodontal abscess (see Chapter 5)
Periodontal-endodontic lesion (see Chapter 5)
Pericoronitis (see Chapter 5)
Dry socket (see Chapter 5)
Sinusitis (see Chapter 6)

2. Viral

Measles
Mumps
Epstein–Barr associated lesions
Human immunodeficiency virus (HIV)
Herpes simplex (see Chapter 10)
Coxsackie (see Chapter 10)
Herpes zoster and chicken pox (see Chapter 6)
Bell's palsy (see Chapter 6)
Cytomegalovirus (CMV) (see Chapter 10)
Human herpes virus 8 (HHV 8) (see Chapter 10)

3. Fungal

Candidiasis/candidosis
Aspergillosis (see Chapter 10)
Histoplasmosis (see Chapter 10)
Mucormycosis (see Chapter 10)
Cryptococcosis (see Chapter 10)
Blastomycosis (see Chapter 10)

Introduction

The major proportion of most dental health care worker's clinical activity is concerned with the diagnosis, treatment and prevention of relevant infections. These can be considered under three headings: bacterial, viral, and fungal.

1. Bacterial

Dental caries

- Progressive, bacterial damage of teeth exposed to the oral environment.
- Is the major cause of tooth loss in young people.
- A complex process of demineralization caused by microbial breakdown of refined carbohydrates.
- Affects the majority of the population in industrialized countries.
- As people retain their teeth for longer, carious attack of the root surface becomes a significant clinical problem.
- Root cementum is particularly vulnerable.
- Not a one way process. Remineralization occurs, particularly in the presence of fluoride.

Caries diagnosis (see also page 27)

- Teeth must be clean, dried and good lighting is essential.
- Every surface of the tooth must be checked for signs of discoloration.
- Margins of restorations must be closely examined for breakdown and leakage.
- Fractured restorations where interproximal amalgam remains in place owing to undercuts in the cavity design, are notorious for developing extensive recurrent caries.
- Particular attention must be given to surfaces that are difficult for patients to clean such as the buccal surfaces of upper third molar teeth and those surfaces which are often neglected, e.g. the lingual surfaces of lower molars.
- Pits, fissures and interproximal surfaces are the most susceptible areas for tooth decay.
- Probes must not be pressed firmly into enamel as this can cause cavitation of the tooth structure and progression of decay.
- Remember also patients who have a high degree of susceptibility to dental caries, e.g. those patients with reduced salivary

flow from drug-induced xerostomia, Sjögren's syndrome or following radiotherapy to the head and neck region.

Symptoms

- Enamel caries does not give rise to symptoms nor does early caries of the dentine.
- More extensive lesions often cause discomfort to patients when eating sweet foods.
- Further progression resulting in inflammatory changes in the pulp, will, if untreated, eventually cause symptoms of pulpitis as described on page 80.

Signs

- White areas of enamel hypocalcification.
- More advanced lesions cause grey/black discoloration.
- Root caries presents as light or dark brown discoloration of root cementum and dentine.
- Active caries of dentine is soft.
- Cavitation.

Diagnostic tests

- There is no substitute for a detailed clinical examination.
- Radiographs, particularly bitewings, are an invaluable diagnostic aid for identifying interproximal lesions and recurrent caries beneath existing restorations.
- The radiographic image of interproximal or occlusal caries, is an 'optimistic' view of the clinical situation and the caries will frequently be seen to be far more extensive when treatment is carried out.
- Vitality tests (see page 35). Thermal, e.g. ice, ethyl chloride, hot gutta percha and electrical.
  Healthy teeth — normal response to hot, cold and electric pulp test.
  Non-vital teeth — no response.
  Pulpitic teeth — early and often excessive response (see also page 36).

N.B. Multi-rooted teeth may give a mixed response which can be difficult to interpret. This is due to the different levels of inflammatory change in different root canals.

Treatment options

1. Prevention — dietary advice, use of fluorides, improve oral hygiene.
2. Observe at regular intervals to monitor remineralization of early lesions and to detect caries progression.

3. Restoration.
4. Extraction.

Osteomyelitis

- Acute or chronic.
- Rare in the developed world.
- Mandible more commonly involved than the maxilla, possibly due to its poorer blood supply and density of the bone.
- May occur following extensive periapical infection.
- May be a consequence of severe facial trauma when bone is exposed, e.g. road traffic accidents, gun shot wounds.
- Acute osteomyelitis may be difficult to differentiate from a dry socket.

Predisposing MH

1. Paget's disease.
2. Previous radiotherapy to the jaws for treatment of neoplasia.
3. Reduced resistance to infection, e.g.
   Immunosuppressant medication
   Acute leukaemia
   Uncontrolled diabetes mellitus
   Chronic alcoholics
   Multiple dietary deficiencies
   Sickle-cell anaemia

Relevant DH

- Apical infection at the time of a tooth extraction.
- Recent extraction of a mandibular tooth under local analgesia, particularly in the presence of ANUG or pericoronitis.
- Apical or lateral periodontitis affecting a tooth in the line of a bony fracture.

Acute osteomyelitis

- Usually due to anaerobic infections by prevotella and fusobacterium species.

Symptoms

- The patient feels unwell and has a raised temperature.
- The jaw is swollen and tender.
- Severe deep-seated pain which is continuous and throbbing.
- Bad taste and discharge of pus into the mouth or onto the face.
- Loose teeth which are painful to bite on.

- Possible numbness of the lower lip.
- Difficulty in opening the mouth.

Signs
- Pyrexia and malaise.
- Intraoral and extraoral sinuses with pus exuding.
- Pus discharging from around the teeth or sockets.
- Swollen face and gingivae.
- Mobile and tender teeth.
- Paraesthesia/anaesthesia of the lip on the affected side.
- Trismus and cervical lymphadenopathy.

Diagnostic tests
- The teeth involved are tender to percussion and give a dull percussion note.
- Test and record any anaesthesia/paraesthesia of the lip or mental region. Use gentle pressure with a dental probe to detect sharp sensation. Use cotton wool strands in college tweezers to assess fine touch.
- Radiographs show ill-defined, often widespread areas of radiolucency with the jaw having a 'moth eaten' appearance. The normal trabecular pattern is lost and when sequestra of dead bone form they appear as more radio-opaque areas. The periodontal ligament space around affected teeth will be widened.
- Bacterial swabs should be taken for culture and sensitivity — a collection of pus is particularly helpful.

Treatment
Refer to hospital for:
- Intravenous antibiotic therapy.
- Debridement and removal of necrotic bone after the acute infection has resolved.

Chronic osteomyelitis
- Less severe symptoms, often asymptomatic.
- May follow an acute episode or occur without an acute phase.
- Sequestra, dead spicules of bone, shed spontaneously.
- Radiographs show considerable sclerosis of adjacent bone and subperiosteal bone formation.

Ludwig's angina

- A severe cellulitis involving the submandibular, sublingual spaces and lateral pharyngeal spaces (Fig. 8.1 and Figs 5.2 and 5.3).

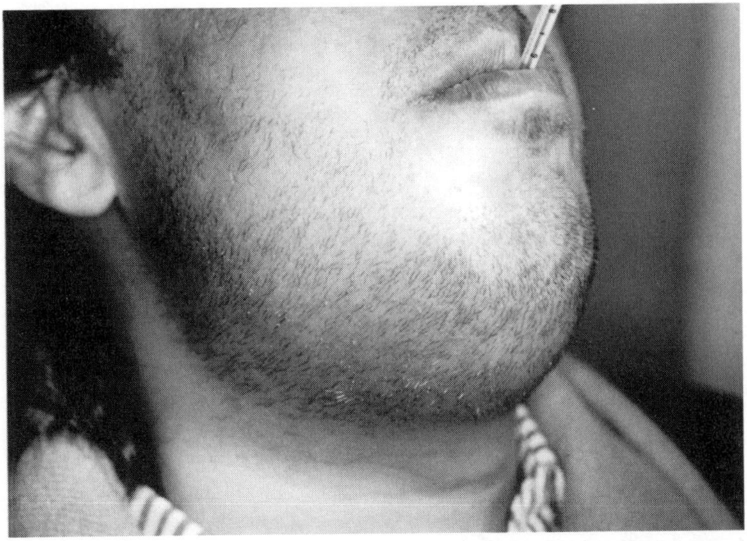

Figure 8.1 Submandibular space infection in a patient with Ludwig's infection.

- Usually caused by streptococci and various mixed anaerobes.
- Infection may spread into the neck via the lateral pharyngeal space.
- Ludwig's angina is a severe, potentially life-threatening infection, as the airway may become progressively restricted. It requires aggressive treatment with intravenous antibiotics.

Symptoms
- Pain and difficulty in swallowing.
- Difficulty in breathing.
- Severe facial pain.
- The patient feels very ill.
- Raised temperature.

Signs
- Rapidly spreading, firm, warm, red, swelling of the face and the neck.
- The tongue is raised, due to the swelling of the floor of the mouth.
- Pyrexia, tachycardia and malaise.
- Difficulty in breathing (stridor), due to oedema of the glottis as well as pressure on the trachea from cellulitis in the neck.

Note: when examining a facial swelling, it is essential to:

1. Record in patient's notes:
Site
Size in mm/cm
Draw diagram or photograph
Note the consistency: **soft** (oedema, abscess, fluid-filled)
firm (cellulitis, lymphadenopathy)
hard (bone-like)

2. Determine whether the swelling is:
Mobile or fixed
Tender on palpation
Warm to touch
Attached to skin or underlying tissue
Assess if fluctuant (Fig. 8.2)

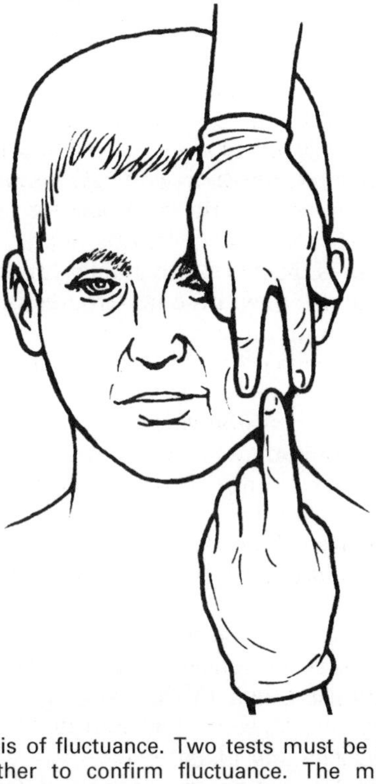

Figure 8.2 Diagnosis of fluctuance. Two tests must be carried out at right angles to each other to confirm fluctuance. The middle finger which depresses the swelling causes fluid to be displaced and this is detected by the two 'watching' fingers at the periphery of the swelling.

Treatment

- Patients must be admitted to hospital for treatment with intravenous antibiotics and incision of the swelling may be required to relieve pressure on the airway.
- The cause, e.g. an infected tooth, must also be established and treated.

Tuberculosis (see also page 189)

- A notifiable disease.
- Worldwide, causes more deaths than any other infectious disease.
- Estimates of the number of people infected as high as 100 million.
- Tuberculosis was in decline in the developed world, but in recent years numbers have begun to increase substantially, *including the UK.*
- The emergence of multi-drug resistant tuberculosis is now a major public health problem particularly in cities such as New York where the situation is further complicated by the increasing prevalance of tuberculosis in patients infected with HIV. Co-infection causes exacerbation of both conditions. Multi-drug resistant tuberculosis has also been reported in small numbers of patients in the UK, including some immigrant groups.
- Rarely there can be persistent oral ulcers, usually on the tongue with undermined borders and a grey/yellow slough, due to local infection.
- Oral tuberculosis generally only arises in patients with active, advanced (open) pulmonary disease.
- Patients receiving anti-tuberculous medication for pulmonary lesions do not have oral changes.
- Oral lesions resolve once patients receive anti-tuberculous medication.
- Tuberculous lymphadenopathy of the cervical lymph nodes (scrofula) particularly common in the Indian subcontinent.

Diagnostic tests

- Biopsy shows caseation (cheese-like consistency), necrosis and multi-nucleated giant cells.
- Presence of mycobacteria can be confirmed by staining for acid fast organisms (Ziehl–Neelsen stain).
- Chest radiography: diffuse mottling of the lungs, cavitation, consolidation and hilar adenopathy.

- Heaf test: rapid exaggerated response.
- Sputum tests: positive for acid-fast bacilli. Can take several weeks to culture.

Syphilis (see also page 189)

- A sexually transmitted disease caused by the spirochaete *Treponema pallidum*.
- A notifiable disease. Referral to a genito-urinary clinic is essential in all suspected cases.
- Relatively rare but must be considered in a differential diagnosis of oral ulceration.
- Can also be passed via the placenta from mother to foetus (congenital syphilis).
- Primary, secondary and tertiary lesions seen in the oral cavity.

For symptoms and signs see page 190.

Primary syphilis

- Rare in the mouth but can occur following direct contact with a lesion (i.e. via orogenital contact).
- Typical oral lesion is a chancre (see page 190).
- They occur approximately 4 weeks after infection.
- Primary lesions of oral syphilis are highly infective.
- Usually heal without scarring after 6–8 weeks.

Secondary syphilis

- Develops 1 to 4 months after the initial infection.
- Causes malaise, headache, mild febrile illness, generalized rash and lymphadenopathy.
- Oral lesions are mucous patches and snail track ulcers (see page 190).
- Ulcers contain large numbers of spirochaetes.

Tertiary syphilis

- Develops several years after the initial infection in untreated cases.
- Oral lesions of tertiary syphilis are gummata and syphilitic leukoplakia (very rare) (see also pages 191, 219).

Gummas

- May grow to a considerable size.
- Are rounded ulcers with punched out edges. They usually occur in the palate and are painless.

Syphilitic leukoplakia

- Seen on the dorsum of the tongue.
- It has a high incidence of malignant transformation.
- Systemic effects of tertiary syphilis include aortitis, tabes dorsalis, dementia and general paresis of the insane (GPI).

Special tests

- Initally in primary syphilis, serology may not be positive.
- Examination of a smear taken from the surface of a chancre will confirm the presence of *T. pallidum* when viewed under dark-ground illumination.
- Serological tests, both non-specific and specific, must be used for screening and diagnosis. They are also important in distinguishing patients with active disease from those who have been effectively treated.
- Non-specific tests: positive in active disease, become negative after treatment:

1. VDRL (Venereal Disease Research Laboratory). N.B. False positive results can occur due to cross-reaction in patients with malaria, viral pneumonia and tuberculosis.
2. RPR (Rapid plasma reagin).

- Specific tests carried out by reference laboratories include:

1. TPHA (*T. pallidum* haemagglutination assay).
2. FTA-Abs (Fluorescent treponemal antibody absorbed test).

Diphtheria

- An infection caused by *Corynebacterium diphtheriae*.
- Rare in the UK.
- Largely eliminated by childhood immunization.
- Increasing incidence in eastern Europe due to the breakdown of vaccination programmes.
- The bacteria produces an exotoxin which can cause myocardial damage and respiratory depression due to nerve paralysis.
- Presents as a grey pseudomembrane on the tonsillar or pharyngeal region.
- Causes difficulty in swallowing.
- Extensive cervical lymph node enlargement occurs.

Actinomycosis

- Usually caused by an oral commensal, *Actinomyces israelii*.
- Pathogenesis unclear.
- A chronic suppurative infection.

- May be a history of oral trauma, e.g. dental extraction, fractured jaw.

Symptoms
- Facial swelling.
- Discharging abscesses on the skin of the face and neck.

Signs
- Chronic indurated abscess, usually at the angle of the mandible.
- Affected skin red/purple colour.
- Multiple sinuses discharging a yellow fluid in which 'sulphur granules' (colonies of the organisms) may be seen.
- May be extensive fibrosis with widespread skin involvement.
- Infection rarely involves the underlying bone.
- Specimen of pus should be sent for culture and antibiotic sensitivity.
- Inform the laboratory actinomycosis is suspected so that appropriate media is used and cultured for a sufficient period of time.

Treatment
Patients with suspected actinomycosis should be referred to hospital for treatment as they may initially require intravenous antibiotics, e.g. penicillin. This is followed by three months of oral therapy with penicillin or amoxycillin. Oral tetracycline is also prescribed to treat the oral flora as this is usually a mixed infection. Abscesses must be drained surgically.

Gram-negative infections in the immunosuppressed patient

- Gram-negative enteric bacteria may cause oropharyngeal infections in the immunocompromised, elderly, the chronically sick and also debilitated patients on long term antibiotic therapy. Organisms include *Escherichia coli*, *Klebsiella* species and *Pseudomonas aeruginosa*.

2. Viral

Measles

- A paramyxovirus spread by droplet infection.
- The incubation period is approximately 10 days.
- Fever, nasal discharge and cough usually present.
- May cause oral lesions termed *Koplik's spots*. These are seen

on the buccal mucosa usually near the molar teeth and are small, white spots on a red base.

- Koplik's spots resolve after 3–4 days to be replaced by a red, maculopapular (see page 22), generalized skin rash.

Mumps

- A paramyxovirus transmitted in saliva.
- A viral infection causing swelling of the salivary glands (sialadenitis).
- Adults may also be affected.
- Incubation period of between 2 to 3 weeks. Patients develop fever, malaise, headache and swelling of the salivary glands, usually the parotids.

Symptoms
- Painful, swollen parotid glands.
- Headache.
- Raised temperature, feel unwell.

Signs
- Pyrexia.
- Unilateral/bilateral tender parotid swellings.
- Other salivary glands — submandibular and sublingual may be involved.

Complications
- Pancreatitis, orchitis (inflammation of the testes), oophoritis (inflammation of the ovaries) and rarely meningitis and encephalitis.

Treatment
- Supportive. Important to ensure adequate levels of hydration.

N.B. Other causes of salivary glands swelling include:

1. Obstructive sialadenitis secondary to calculus formation.
2. Acute ascending parotitis in xerostomia (dry mouth).
3. The salivary glands may also be enlarged in conditions such as Sjögren's syndrome, sarcoidosis and salivary gland tumours.

Epstein–Barr virus

- A human herpesvirus, found in latent form in more than 90% of the population.

- Primary infection may be subclinical, or give rise to infectious mononucleosis (glandular fever).
- Causes oral hairy leukoplakia in immunosupressed patients.
- EBV can be found in the saliva of asymptomatic seropositive individuals as well as those with clinical symptoms.

Symptoms of infectious mononucleosis

- Usually in adolescents.
- Sore throat.
- Tiredness, feel unwell.
- Headaches.
- Swollen lymph glands.
- Rarely mouth ulcers.
- Abdominal pain (due to hepatic and splenic involvement).
- Muscle pain (myalgia).

Signs

- Pyrexia.
- Cevical lymph nodes enlarged.
- Oral ulceration — usually the posterior region of the mouth and the pharynx.
- Petechiae (small discrete blood-filled macules or papules) on the soft palate.
- Pharyngitis.
- Skin rash.

N.B. Ampicillin and amoxycillin also cause a generalized maculopapular rash when given to patients with infectious mononucleosis.

Diagnostic tests

- Full blood count reveals an atypical lymphocytosis and occasional thrombocytopenia.
- Paul–Bunnell or Monospot blood test, to determine the prescence of heterophile antibodies.
- Occasional assessment of liver function may be appropriate.
- Paul–Bunnell negative, glandular fever-like disorders, include HIV, cytomegalovirus and toxoplasma infection.
- Treatment is symptomatic. Antimicrobial mouthwashes can relieve intraoral symptoms.
- Epstein–Barr virus is also associated with Burkitt's lymphoma, nasopharyngeal carcinoma and oral hairy leukoplakia.

Human immunodeficiency virus (HIV)

- An RNA virus which infects T4 helper cells (also known as CD4+ T lymphocytes).

- Causes progressive impairment of the immune system, resulting in opportunistic infections.
- Oral opportunistic infection may be the first sign of HIV disease.
- More than 50 oral manifestations of HIV disease have been described and up to 90% of patients with HIV disease have changes in and around the oral cavity.
- **Oral manifestations of HIV are now classified according to the degree of their association with HIV infection:**

Group 1 Lesions strongly asssociated with HIV infection

- Candidiasis — erythematous, pseudomembranous
- Hairy leukoplakia
- Periodontal diseases — Linear gingival erythema
  Necrotizing ulcerative gingivitis
  Necrotizing ulcerative periodontitis
- Kaposi's sarcoma
- Non-Hodgkin's lymphoma

Group 2 Lesions less commonly associated with HIV infection

- Bacterial infections
  - *Mycobacterium avium intracellulare*
  - *Mycobacterium tuberculosis*
- Melanotic hyperpigmentation
- Necrotizing (ulcerative) stomatitis
- Ulceration (not otherwise specified)
- Salivary gland disease
  - Dry mouth due to decreased salivary flow
  - Unilateral or bilateral swelling of major salivary glands
- Thrombocytopenic purpura
- Viral infections
  - HSV (herpes simplex virus)
  - HPV (human papilloma virus)
  - Condyloma acuminatum
  - Focal epithelial hyperplasia
  - Verruca vulgaris
  - Varicella zoster
  - Herpes zoster

Group 3 Lesions seen in HIV infection
(Previously 'Lesions possibly associated with HIV')

- Bacterial infections
  - *Actinomyces israelii*
  - *Escherichia coli*
  - *Klebsiella pneumoniae*

Continued

Mycobacterium avium intracellulare
Mycobacterium tuberculosis
- Cat scratch disease
- Drug reactions (ulcerative, erythema multiforme, lichenoid, toxic epidermolysis)
- Fungal infections other than candidiasis
  Cryptococcus neoformans
  Geotrichum candidum
  Histoplasma capsulatum
  Mucoraceae (Mucormycosis)
  Aspergillus flavus
- Neurologic disturbances
  Facial palsy
  Trigeminal neuralgia
- Recurrent aphthous stomatitis
- Viral infections
  Cytomegalovirus
  Molluscum contagiosum

- The dental team has an important role in the early recognition of these oral changes.
- Early identification enables the patient to receive prompt appropriate medical care and counselling, increasing life expectancy and helping to reduce further spread of the disease.

3. Fungal

Candidiasis (candidosis)

Candidiasis and candidosis are synonymous. Many recently published texts refer to candidosis but the WHO preferred term candidiasis will be used here.
- Candidal species are found as oral commensals in up to 90% of the population.
- *Candida albicans* is the most frequently isolated strain.
- Clinical infection occurs with immunosuppression, xerostomia and altered oral microflora concentrations, e.g. following use of broad spectrum antibiotics.

Predisposing factors include:
- Denture wearing.
- Reduced salivation, e.g. drug-induced.

- Antibiotic therapy, particularly broad spectrum agents.
- Poorly controlled diabetes mellitus.
- Corticosteroid therapy (including inhalers taken for asthma).
- Radiotherapy to the oral region and resultant salivary gland damage.
- Iron, vitamin B_{12} and folic acid deficiencies.
- Immunosuppression including:
  1. HIV
  2. Leukaemia
  3. Agranulocytosis
  4. Cytotoxic drugs
  5. Malnutrition and malabsorption

Clinical candidiasis presents as:

1. Acute candidiasis

a. Pseudomembranous (thrush) (Fig. 8.3).

Symptoms

- May be asymptomatic.
- Can cause a sore, painful mouth.
- Discomfort on swallowing.

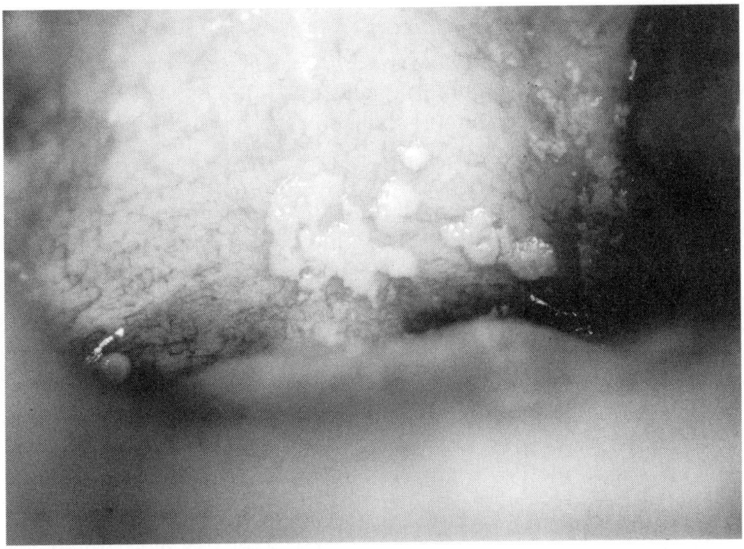

Figure 8.3 Pseudomembranous candidiasis.

Signs
- Pseudomembranous candidiasis presents as creamy, white/yellow patches on the oral mucosa which can be removed easily, leaving behind an erythematous, sometimes bleeding, surface.

b. Atrophic (erythematous).
- Seen in patients on steroid therapy and broad spectrum antibiotics.

Symptoms
- Often painful.

Signs
- Red, inflamed mucosa. Any site may be involved, including the palate, tongue and buccal mucosa.
- Erythematous candidiasis, seen in HIV positive patients is essentially a chronic condition.
- It presents as red areas, usually on the palate and on the dorsum of the tongue. In HIV positive patients the classic appearance of erythematous candidiasis is that of a central area of erythema in the palate with normal tissue adjacent to the gingival margin. The so called 'thumb print' appearance (Figs 8.4 and 8.5).

2. Chronic atrophic candidiasis (chronic erythematous candidiasis, denture-induced stomatitis, denture sore mouth)
- Coverage of the palatal mucosa for lengthy periods by a denture or orthodontic appliance is the predisposing factor.

Symptoms
- Usually symptom-free.

Signs
- Erythematous inflamed mucosa.
- Corresponds to the area of the palate covered by either a denture or orthodontic applicance.
- Mucosa not covered by the prosthesis is healthy in appearance.
- 'Denture sore mouth' is a misnomer as patients are often unaware of its presence.
- The commonest presentation of candidal infection with an incidence of between 25 and 50% in denture wearers.

N.B. The *denture itself* is also colonized by candidal organisms which can reinfect the palate.

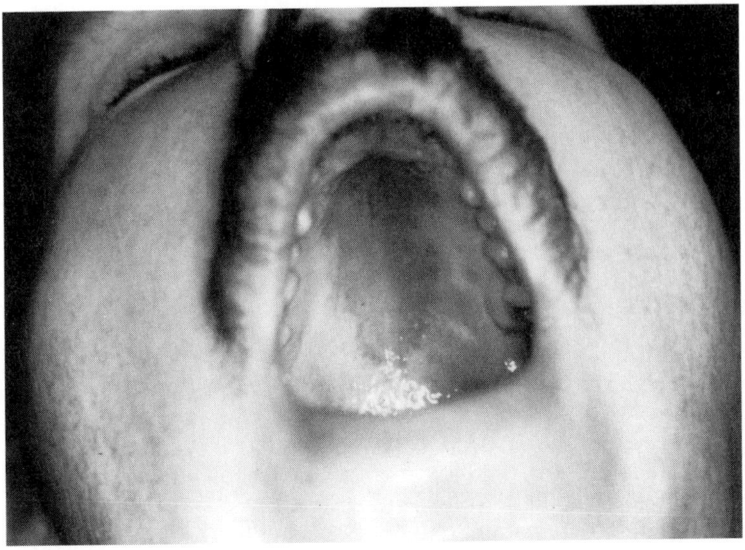

Figure 8.4 Erythematous candidiasis ('thumb print' on palate).

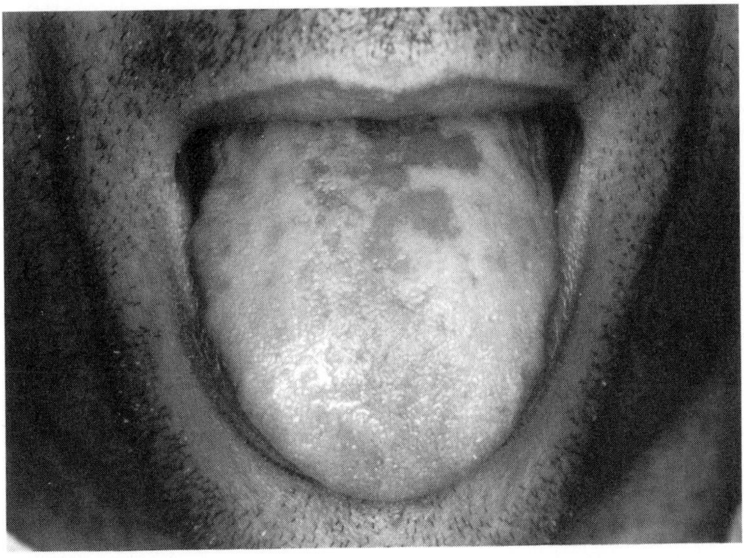

Figure 8.5 Erythematous candidiasis on dorsum of tongue in an HIV positive patient.

Treatment should include
- Advising patients to leave their dentures out when asleep at night.
- Ensuring that dentures are scrupulously clean and soaked overnight in a solution of chlorhexidine or hypochlorite.
- Ill-fitting dentures must be replaced once the inflammatory changes have resolved.
- The use of tissue conditioners to improve the fit of the dentures during this period is advisable.
- Topical antifungals, e.g. nystatin, amphotericin B and chlorhexidine mouthwash may be prescribed.
- Patients should coat the fitting surface of their denture with miconazole gel before insertion.

NB. Warfarin therapy contraindicates the use of miconazole.

3. Angular cheilitis (stomatitis)
- Associated with loss of vertical dimension and lower facial height, in patients with worn dentures.
- In the dentate patient may be associated with vitamin B_{12}, folic acid or iron deficiency.
- Is a feature of immunosuppression, particularly HIV disease and neutropenias.

Symptoms
- Sore, painful corners of the mouth.

Signs
- Cracked, inflamed skin folds at the angles of the mouth.
- May accompany intraoral candidiasis.
- Bacteria, e.g. staphylococcal organisms, can also cause angular cheilitis.

Treatment
- Includes identifying the cause of and eliminating any underlying blood deficiency states.
- Replacement of worn dentures and establishment of the correct vertical dimension.
- Treatment of any associated intra-oral candidal infection.
- Topical antimicrobial medication.

4. Chronic hyperplastic candidiasis (candidal leukoplakia)
See page 218

5. Chronic mucocutaneous candidiasis
- Oral candidal infection can also occur as part of rare mucocutaneous disorders, e.g.

a. Familial (limited). Inherited as an autosomal recessive trait.
b. Diffuse (sporadic). Rare familial cases.
c. Late onset (thymoma syndrome). Defect of cell-mediated immunity caused by a thymoma.
d. Endocrine (candidiasis-endocrinopathy syndrome). Multiple glandular deficiencies, e.g. hypoparathyroidism or Addison's disease and autoantibody production.

Diagnostic tests

- A smear from the affected region should be taken and stained (Gram's stain or PAS (periodic acid-Schiff) reagent). Potassium hydroxide (KOH) can also be applied to a smear to demonstrate hyphae.
- A swab and an oral rinse should also be taken and sent for culture.
- Quantitative candidal counts may be useful as the response to therapy can be monitored. Patients should provide a sample of saliva or rinse and gargle with phosphate-buffered saline for one minute before expectorating into a sterile container.
- Biopsy and histopathological examination is necessary to confirm chronic hyperplastic candidiasis.

The 'deep' mycoses (See p. 195)

- Aspergillosis
- Histoplasmosis
- Mucormycosis
- Cryptococcosis
- Blastomycosis

Further reading

Cawson, R.A. (1991) *Essentials of Dental Surgery and Pathology*, 5th edn. Edinburgh: Churchill Livingstone.

Glick, M. (1994) *Dental Management of Patients with HIV*. Chicago: Quintessence.

Marsh, P. and Martin, M. (1992) *Oral Microbiology*, 3rd edn. London: Chapman and Hall.

Scully, C. and Cawson, R.A. (1998) *Medical Problems in Dentistry*, 4th edn. Oxford: Wright.

Tyldesley, W.R. and Field, E.A. (1995) *Oral Medicine*, 4th edn. Oxford: Oxford University Press.

Cysts

Summary

Definition
Introduction
History of present complaint
Symptoms
Signs
Classification
(World Health Organization Publication *Histological Typing of Odontogenic Tumours*. Kramer, Pindborg and Shear, l992, Modified by Shear)

I. Cysts of the jaws

Epithelial

Developmental

(a) Odontogenic
1. Gingival cyst of infants
2. Odontogenic keratocyst (primordial cyst)
3. Dentigerous (follicular) cyst
4. Eruption cyst
5. Lateral periodontal cyst
6. Gingival cyst of adults
7. Botryoid odontogenic cyst
8. Glandular odontogenic cyst

(Sialo-odontogenic mucoepidermoid odontogenic cyst)

(b) Non-odontogenic
1. Nasopalatine duct (incisive canal) cyst
2. Nasolabial (nasoalveolar cyst)
3. Median palatine, median alveolar, median mandibular cysts
4. Globulomaxillary cyst

Epithelial

Inflammatory
1. Radicular cyst, apical and lateral
2. Residual cyst
3. Paradental cyst and mandibular infected buccal cyst
4. Inflammatory collateral cyst

Non-epithelial
1. Solitary bone cyst (traumatic, simple, haemorrhagic bone cyst)
2. Aneurysmal bone cyst

continued

II. Cysts associated with the maxillary antrum
1. Benign mucosal cyst of the maxillary antrum
2. Postoperative maxillary cyst (surgical ciliated cyst of the maxilla)

III. Cyst of the soft tissues of the mouth, face and neck
1. Dermoid and epidermoid cysts
2. Lympho-epithelial (branchial cleft cyst)
3. Thyroglossal duct cyst
4. Anterior median lingual cyst (intralingual cyst of foregut origin)
5. Oral cysts with gastric or intestinal epithelium (oral alimentary tract cyst)
6. Cystic hygroma
7. Nasopharyngeal cysts
8. Thymic cyst
9. Cysts of the salivary glands, mucous extravasation cyst, mucous retention cyst, ranula, polycystic (dysgenetic) disease of the parotid
10. Parasitic cysts, hydatid cysts, cysticercus cellulosae, trichinosis

Definition

A cyst is a pathological cavity with fluid, semi-fluid or gaseous contents and which is not created by the accumulation of pus. It is frequently, but not always, lined by epithelium.
The epithelium in odontogenic and inflammatory cysts of the jaws is derived from:

- the tooth germ, or
- the reduced enamel epithelium, or
- the epithelial rest cells of Malassez, or
- remnants of the dental lamina

Introduction

Cysts are usually painless when small and can cause significant bone loss before becoming detectable clinically.

As with other oral conditions a comprehensive history is required. This begins with:

History of present complaint

Ask your patient:

- Are you in pain? (dull and throbbing with infected cyst).
- Do you have a swollen face/mouth? Is the swelling increasing/decreasing in size?
- Any toothache or loose teeth?
- Any discoloured teeth?
- A bad taste?
- Do your dentures still fit?
- Is your bite altered?
- Have any teeth moved?

Symptoms

- Generally painless when the cyst is small.
- Often discovered by chance on radiographs taken for other reasons.
- Frequently symptom free—even large cysts.
- Pain and swelling occur when the cyst becomes infected.
- May have a swelling, either intra or extraorally, e.g. lump in the labial/buccal sulcus or swelling in the palate.
- Infected cysts may discharge intraorally causing an unpleasant taste.
- In the edentulous or partially dentate patient, expansion of the alveolus by the cyst may displace a denture or lead to ulceration of the mucosa.
- Gaps appearing between teeth (enlarging cysts may displace teeth).
- A discoloured tooth may be the patient's presenting complaint (discoloration and loss of vitality may be associated with a radicular cyst).
- Loosening of teeth.
- Altered bite—with pathological fractures.
- Numbness of the lower lip (infected cyst, pathological fracture).
- Trismus (limited jaw opening, infected cyst, pathological fracture).

N.B. Large cysts may cause pathological fractures with disturbance of occlusion as well as pain.

They may also cause pressure on the inferior dental nerve with associated labial paraesthesia.

Signs

- Can be extremely variable.
- Small cysts may cause no discernible change.

- Check for missing teeth from an otherwise complete arch, e.g. dentigerous, eruption and odontogenic keratocysts.
- Non-vital teeth may be discoloured.
- Large cysts can cause expansion of the alveolar bone.
- Initially there is bony hard expansion of the jaw.
- Ultimately, thinning of the cortex occurs.
- Palpation then causes 'egg-shell crackling' (gentle finger pressure on the bone surface produces the sounds and sensation of breaking egg shells).

- When no bone covers a cyst, and the lining is in contact with mucosa a bluish colour is seen, together with fluctuance. (For test for fluctuance see p. 146.)
- Cysts of the soft tissues of the mouth cause visible and palpable swellings.
- May displace teeth or give rise to increased mobility.
- Teeth remain vital apart from apical and lateral radicular cysts.
- Sinuses may be present if the cyst has discharged into the oral cavity.
- Abnormal mandibular mobility and altered occlusion, occur with pathological fractures.

Diagnostic tests include

- Radiography both intra- and extraoral.
- Cysts appear as radiolucencies surrounded by a clearly defined, white, radiopaque, sclerotic margin.
- Vitality testing — unless associated with radicular cysts, teeth remain vital.
- Sialography, for salivary gland cysts.
- Aspiration of fluid contents:
  Straw-coloured fluid containing cholesterol crystals obtained from most *radicular cysts*.
  Air, some blood or serosanguineous fluid from *solitary bone cysts*.
  Blood from *aneurysmal bone cyst*.
  Pus from *infected cysts*.
  Pale, yellow fluid containing keratin from *odontogenic keratocyst*.
- Biopsy of lining, provides definitive diagnosis.

It is essential to send all soft tissue removed at surgery for histological examination.

Although rare, the literature does contain well documented, reported cases of squamous cell carcinoma arising from the epithelial lining of odontogenic cysts. Shear (1992) states, however, that in view of the extreme rarity of such change, *there is no evidence to consider cysts as pre-cancerous lesions*, although tumours can mimic the radiological features of some cysts, e.g. ameloblastomas can mimic odontogenic keratocysts.

I. Cysts of the jaw

Epithelial

Developmental

(a) Odontogenic

1. Gingival cysts of infants

Aetiology
- Derived from remnants of the dental lamina.

Symptoms
- Symptomless, soft-tissue swellings, on alveolar ridges.

Signs
- Rarely seen after 3 months of age.
- Can occur singly or more commonly, several are present. White or cream coloured in appearance.
- Disappear without treatment.

They are disrupted by tooth eruption and can rupture through the surface of the mucosa.

- Also known as Bohn's nodules or Epstein's pearls.

2. Odontogenic keratocyst (primordial cyst) (Figs 9.1 and 9.2)
- Now recognized as a distinct clinical entity.
- Peak incidence in the second and third decades.
- Accounts for between 8 and 11% of odontogenic cysts.
- Multiple odontogenic keratocysts and basal cell carcinomas are seen in naevoid basal cell carcinoma syndrome, also known as Gorlin and Goltz syndrome, an inherited autosomal, dominant condition.
- High incidence of recurrence after surgical treatment.
- May mimic other lesions, e.g. lateral periodontal cyst.
- Potential for aggressive growth.

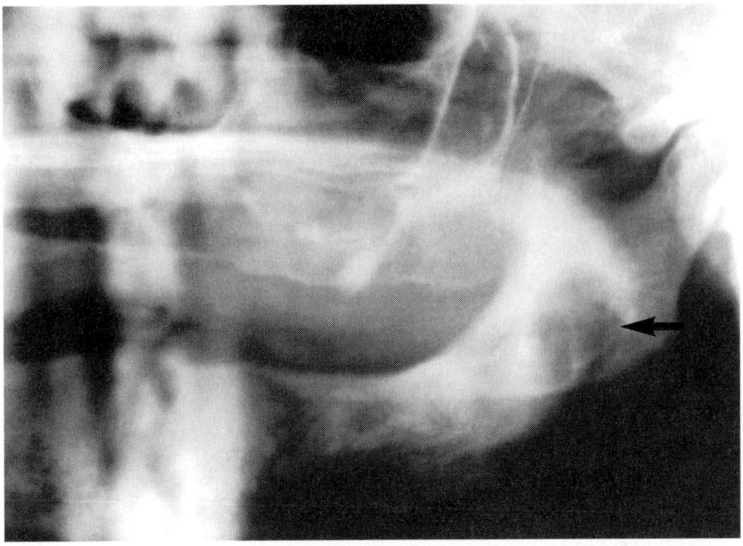

Figure 9.1 Recurrent odontogenic keratocyst in the left ascending ramus.

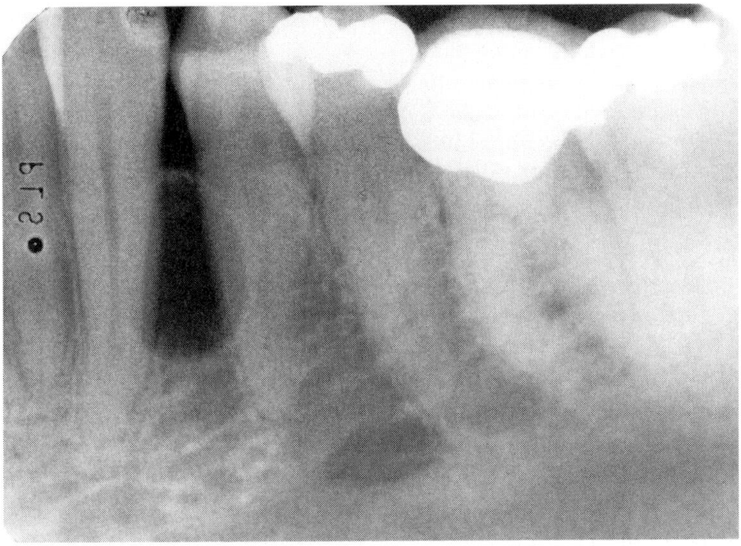

Figure 9.2 Odontogenic keratocyst mimicking a lateral periodontal cyst.

Symptoms

- Small cysts often symptom-free unless infected.
- Then cause pain, swelling and discharge.
- Numbness of the lower lip when infected or when pathological fracture has occurred.
- Can become extensive involving the entire ascending ramus including the condyle and coronoid processes without causing symptoms.
- Has a tendency to grow in the medullary cavity of bone and expansion occurs late.

Diagnostic tests

Radiography

- Majority are unilocular radiolucencies, with radiopaque sclerotic margins.
- Some have scalloped margins and may be misinterpreted as multilocular lesions.
- Most common in the mandible, particularly the molar and ramus regions.
- Multilocular odontogenic keratocysts do occur.
- And may be indistinguishable from an ameloblastoma on radiograph.
- Root resorption rarely occurs.

Biopsy

- Provides definitive diagnosis.
- Histology is characteristic.
- The cysts are thin walled, ortho- or parakeratinized with satellite cysts seen (up to 50%) in the capsular fibrous tissue.
- Aspiration:- lumen contains pale yellow fluid with desquamated keratin.

3. Dentigerous (follicular) cyst (Fig. 9.3)

- Caused by expansion of the dental follicle.
- Encloses the crown of an unerupted tooth.

Symptoms

- Like other cysts, painful when infected.
- Can remain symptom free in spite of growing to a large size.

Signs

- Expansion of the alveolus when large.

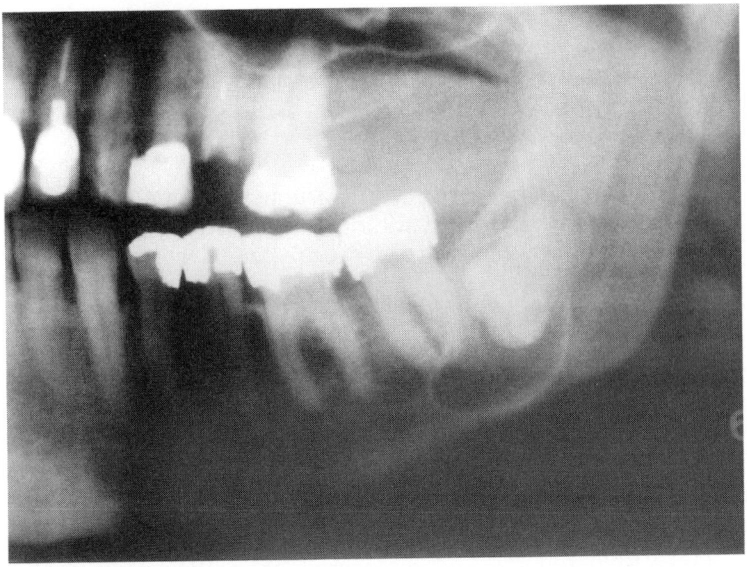

Figure 9.3 Dentigerous cyst.

- Majority are associated with unerupted, mandibular third molars.
- May cause tilting of the adjacent teeth.

Diagnostic tests

Radiographs

- Appears as a unilocular radiolucent area associated with the crown of an unerupted tooth.
- Cysts have well-defined sclerotic margins.
- The cyst encloses the crown (and is attached to the neck) of the tooth.
- Root resorption of adjacent teeth may occur.

4. Eruption cyst

- Rare.
- A superficial cyst occurring in the gingival tissues.
- Associated with an erupting tooth most commonly the deciduous molars.

Symptoms
- Painless unless infected.
- May be pain on biting if there is an opposing tooth.
- Swollen gum.

Signs
- Presents as a gingival swelling which may be blue in colour.
- Swelling is soft and fluctuant.
- May burst spontaneously or can be treated by marsupialization, exposing the crown of the tooth which can then erupt.

Diagnostic tests
Radiography confirms an unerupted tooth, with an enlarged follicle.

5. *Lateral periodontal cyst*
- Arising from the epithelial remnants in the periodontal ligament.

Symptoms
- Pain, gingival tenderness and swelling.
- Often symptomless and discovered on routine radiographic examination.

Signs
- Usually seen in the mandibular canine and premolar region.
- Teeth are vital.

Radiographs
- Round radiolucency associated with the lateral surface of a tooth.
- Surrounded by a well-demarcated cortical margin.
- No root resorption.
- Indistinguishable radiographically from keratocysts.
- Definitive diagnosis is made by histological examination.

6. *Gingival cyst of adults*
- Rare. Very few cases reported.
- Most occurring between the ages of 40 and 60.

Symptoms
- Painless swelling on the gum.

Signs
- A gingival swelling usually in the lower premolar and canine region on the buccal aspect.
- Soft and fluctuant.

- When removed by surgical excision, slight indentation on the underlying bone may be seen.
- Do not tend to recur.

Diagnostic tests
- Biopsy: confirms the diagnosis.
- Radiography: no change.

7. Botryoid odontogenic cyst
- Considered to be a variant of lateral periodontal cysts.

Symptoms
- Pain and swelling when infected.

Signs
- Majority of lesions are seen in the mandible.
- Tender alveolar swelling.

Diagnostic tests
Radiology
- Multilocular radiolucencies.

Biopsy
- Multilocular, macroscopically resembling a 'bunch of grapes', hence the name.
- Have a tendency to recur and long-term follow-up after treatment is essential.

8. Glandular odontogenic cyst
- Very rare.
- Resembles the botryoid odontogenic cyst.

Diagnostic tests
- May be unilocular or multilocular on radiographic examination, with smooth cortical margin.

In view of the multilocular appearance and tendency to recur, long-term follow-up, after treatment, is also essential.

(b) Non-odontogenic

1. Nasopalatine duct (incisive canal) cyst
- The most common non-odontogenic cyst.

- Caused by proliferation of epithelial remnants within the nasopalatine canal.

Symptoms
- Many are asymptomatic.
- Most common symptom is a swelling in the midline of the palate behind the upper central incisor teeth.
- Labial swelling may also occur with or without the palatal swelling.
- May cause pain particularly when secondary infection occurs.
- May discharge with a salty or foul taste.

Signs

- May be no changes.
- Tender palatal or labial swelling adjacent to the upper incisor teeth.
- Displacement of the incisors may occur but teeth remain vital.

Diagnostic tests
Biopsy provides definitive diagnosis. Cysts are lined by a combination of stratified squamous, cuboidal and ciliated columnar epithelium.

Aspiration: pus when infected.

Radiology
- A circular well circumscribed radiolucency between 1|1.
- The upper standard occlusal radiograph is useful to demonstrate the presence of an intact lamina dura around the upper incisor teeth.
- A radiographic shadow of the incisive canal less than 6 mm wide can be considered to be within normal limits in the absence of specific symptoms but in negroid skulls a width of as much as 10 mm in the incisive fossa region may be normal.
- In the absence of other symptoms or signs, these patients should be observed and repeat radiographs taken at regular intervals, e.g. annually.

2. *Nasolabial (nasoalveolar) cyst*
A rare soft tissue cyst more common in females.

Symptoms
- Swollen lip.
- Pain free unless secondarily infected.

Signs
- Presents as a swelling of the lip, raising the alar cartilages.
- Extends into the floor of the nose and labial sulcus.
- Fluctuant.

Diagnostic tests
Aspiration
- Straw-coloured mucinous fluid. No cholesterol crystals.
- Pus when infected.

Radiology
- Standard occlusal radiograph shows a posterior convexity in one half of the bracket shaped line which forms the border of the nasal aperture.
- Differential diagnosis includes an alveolar abscess from an upper anterior tooth.
- Pulp testing of the upper anteriors (they are vital) is required to confirm the diagnosis.

3. Median palatine, median alveolar, median mandibular cysts

Median palatine and median alveolar cysts:
- Histological features are identical to the nasopalatine duct cyst.
- They are now considered to be either posterior extensions of the nasopalatine duct cyst in the case of median palatine cyst or anterior extensions in the case of the median alveolar cyst.

Median mandibular cysts occur, as the name suggests, in the midline of the mandible

Symptoms
- Symptom free.
- Pain when infected.
- Swelling in the mental region.
- Gaps between lower incisor teeth.

Signs
- Firm or fluctuant mandibular swelling in the incisor region.
- When large can cause displacement of the lower incisor teeth which remain vital.

Diagnostic tests
Radiology
- Circumscribed radiolucency.

Biopsy

- Histological examination of many of the 'reported cases', confirm diagnoses of either *keratocysts or solitary bone cysts.*

Little evidence, then, that the median mandibular cyst is a distinct entity.

4. Globulomaxillary cyst

Symptoms

- Usually symptom free.

Signs

- Found on radiograph between the upper lateral incisor and canine teeth.
- Expansion causes displacement of the root apices and convergence of the crowns of the teeth.
- Teeth remain vital.
- No longer thought to be a fissural cyst caused by inclusion of non odontogenic epithelium during the embryological development of the maxilla.
- Now considered to be various odontogenic cysts and tumours, e.g. odontogenic keratocysts, radicular cysts and lateral periodontal cysts. Other lesions such as ameloblastomas, solitary bone cysts and odontogenic myxomas have also been reported in the incisor/canine region and *misdiagnosed* as globulomaxillary cysts.

Diagnostic tests

- Radiology: a well defined radiolucency between 2|2 and 3|3.
- Vitality tests: teeth remain vital except for radicular cysts.
- Biopsy provides a definitive diagnosis.
- Differential diagnosis includes lateral periodontal cysts, keratocysts, giant cell granulomas, ameloblastomas, myxomas and solitary bone cysts.

Epithelial

Inflammatory

1. Radicular cysts (apical and lateral)

- The most common cystic lesion in the jaws; develops from proliferation of epithelial cell remnants in the periodontal ligament *(cell rests of Malassez).*
- These are stimulated by the inflammatory products which occur following the death of a dental pulp.

- Following the extraction of the causative tooth, if the cyst is overlooked, it can continue to develop and is termed a **residual cyst (2)**.

Symptoms
- Radicular cysts may be asymptomatic and found on routine dental radiography.
- Pain and swelling occur when infected.
- Purulent discharge and unpleasant taste if the swelling drains spontaneously.
- Discoloured teeth due to loss of vitality.

Signs
- As cysts enlarge, hard swellings may appear intraorally, either buccally or lingually.
- Further expansion erodes the bone and fluctuance may be present.
- Associated teeth are tender to percussion, when cysts are infected.
- Teeth are non-vital, discoloured and may show increased mobility.
- May be retained roots present.

Diagnostic tests
Radiology
- A radiolucency with a well circumscribed cortical margin which may be lost following infection.

Aspiration
- Straw coloured fluid containing cholesterol crystals.
- Pus present when infected.
- Biopsy for definitive histological diagnosis.

3. Paradental and mandibular infected buccal cyst
- *Paradental cyst* (Fig. 9.4): an inflammatory cyst seen on the lateral aspect of a tooth. It is caused by inflammation in a periodontal *pocket* and stimulation of the epithelial rest cells of Malassez or the reduced enamel epithelium. (Paradental cysts are associated with partially erupted third molars.)
- *Mandibular infected buccal cyst* considered to be a variety of the paradental cyst, occurring in relation to the mandibular first and second molars in children.

Symptoms
- Can be symptom free.

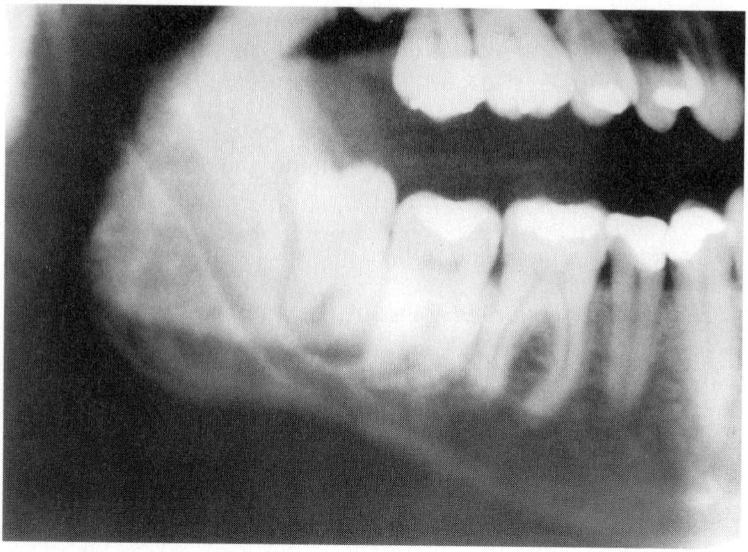

Figure 9.4 Paradental cyst, 8⏋.

- May cause pain, tenderness and swelling if infected.
- Symptoms can be more severe in children.
- Facial swelling and facial sinus may occur.

Signs
- Tooth is partially erupted.
- Cyst occurs on the buccal surface. There may be buccal expansion.
- Teeth remain vital.

Diagnostic tests
- Radiology: radiolucency present. Affected tooth tilted. New bone may be laid down.
- Lamina dura intact.
- Biopsy : indistinguishable from a radicular cyst histologically.
- Aspiration: pus obtained when infected.

4. Inflammatory collateral cyst
- An inflammatory cyst of the gingiva.
- Aetiology: inflammation in a periodontal pocket causing proliferation of rest cells of Malassez.

- Rare.
- Seen on erupted teeth (paradental cysts occur on partially erupted teeth).

Symptoms
- May be symptom free.
- Painful gingival swelling.

Signs
- Teeth remain vital.
- Periodontal disease.

Non-epithelial

1. Solitary bone cyst *(traumatic, simple, haemorrhagic bone cyst)* (Fig. 9.5)

Aetiology
- Unknown.

Thought to be caused by trauma which causes intramedullary haemorrage. Failure of the clot to organize and its subsequent

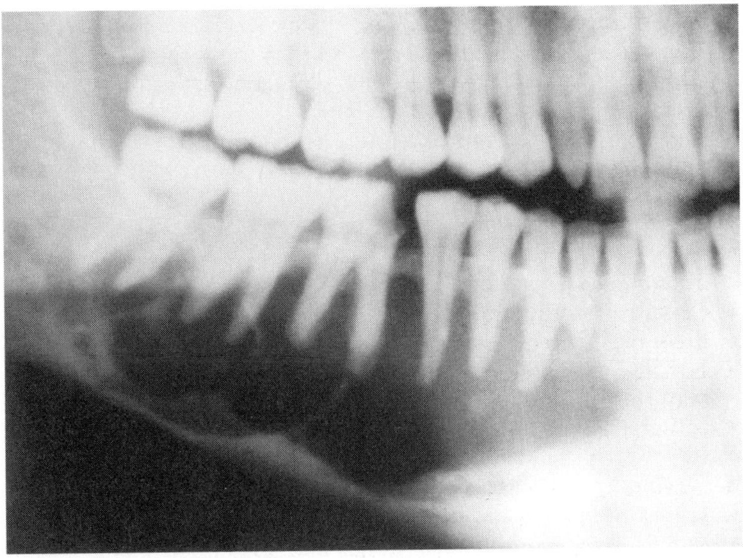

Figure 9.5 Solitary bone cyst.

degeneration leads to the production of an empty cavity within the bone.

Symptoms
- The majority are symptom free and discovered by chance on routine radiography.
- Symptoms, when present, include pain, swelling and paraesthesia.

Signs
- Mandibular swelling.
- Rarely seen in the maxilla.
- Most patients are young in the second decade of life.

Diagnostic tests
Radiology
- Unilocular radiolucency but scalloping may appear between teeth and between the roots of molars.
- The roots of adjacent teeth not usually resorbed.
- Vitality tests: teeth remain vital.

Aspiration
- Usually devoid of fluid contents and contain air or nitrogen.
- Some contain blood clot or serosanguineous fluid with high concentration of bilirubin.
- The differential diagnosis of a solitary bone cyst from other cysts of the jaws may therefore be made clinically by aspiration.
- At surgery these cysts are found to be empty and without an epithelial lining.
- Spontaneous regression may occur.

2. *Aneurysmal bone cyst*
- Unknown aetiology. Little evidence to support a trauma theory.
- Possibly a secondary phenomenon arising in a pre-existing bone lesion, e.g. ossifying fibroma, fibrous dysplasia or giant cell granuloma.
- Rare in the jaws though can occur in both the mandible and maxilla.
- Found in all parts of the skeleton.
- Majority occur in the long bones and spine.
- Seen mainly in children and adults under 30 years of age.

Symptoms
- Usually painless swellings of the jaw.

Signs
- Swellings are firm.
- There is displacement of teeth and malocclusion.
- May be egg-shell crackling.

Diagnostic tests
The teeth remain vital.

Radiology
- A unilocular or multilocular radiolucency.
- Described as either a *'blow out'* or *'soap bubble'* appearance.
- Root resorption may occur.
- High recurrence rate following treatment.

II. Cysts associated with the maxillary antrum

1. Benign mucosal cyst of the maxillary antrum
- Also known as a mucocele or retention cyst.

Symptoms
- Many cases are found on routine panoramic radiography and are asymptomatic.
- Rarely symptoms may include nasal obstruction and discharge or a dull pain in the antral region.

Diagnostic tests
Radiology
- Cysts appear as spherical radiopacities with a smooth, uniform outline.
- There is no resorption of the adjacent bone.
- Most remain static or regress spontaneously.
- More frequent diagnosis nowadays with increased use of panoramic radiographs.
- Differential diagnosis includes inflammatory conditions of the maxillary sinus, e.g. apical radicular cysts, postoperative maxillary cysts and superimposition of normal anatomy such as the nasal conchae.

2. Postoperative maxillary cyst

- Commonly encountered in Japan but rare in other parts of the world.
- It is a delayed complication often arising several years after surgery involving the maxillary sinus.
- Seen following antral surgery, particularly the Caldwell–Luc procedure.
- Can also occur from gunshot injuries and fractures of the mid-face.

Symptoms

- Pain and swelling of the cheek or face.

Signs

- Intraoral swelling may also be seen with discharge of pus.
- As cysts enlarge, the sinus wall may become thinned or even perforate.

Diagnostic tests

Radiology

- Radiographs confirm a well-defined radiolucent area related to the maxillary sinus.
- Most are unilocular with surrounding bony sclerosis.
- Differential diagnosis includes malignant tumours as expansion can lead to perforation of the antral wall.

Histology

- Cysts are lined with pseudostratified ciliated columnar epithelium.

III. Cysts of the soft tissues of the mouth, face and neck

1. Dermoid and epidermoid cysts

Aetiology:

- Developmental, derived from embryonic epithelium trapped during closure of the mandibular arches.
- Dermoid and epidermoid cysts may occur on the floor of the mouth.
- Can be present at birth.
- The majority are seen between the ages of 15 and 35 years.

- Most common site is the midline of the floor of the mouth
- Also occur on the face.

Symptoms
- Patient may present with difficulty in speaking, eating, breathing or closing the mouth.

Signs
- A midline swelling which raises the tongue.
- The swelling may extend into the neck giving the patient a double chin appearance.
- Soft to palpation.

Diagnostic tests
Biopsy
- Lined by epidermis.
- The dermoid cyst contains skin appendages in the fibrous wall.

Radiology: no changes.

Vitality tests: normal response.
- Differential diagnoses include ranula, sublingual space infection and cellulitis from a spreading dental abscess.

2. *Lympho-epithelial (branchial cleft) cyst*

Aetiology
- Developmental, derived from epithelial remnants of the branchial arches and pharyngeal pouches or may represent cystic change of salivary gland epithelium trapped in cervical lymph nodes.
- Occur on the lateral aspect of the neck, in the parotid gland and in the mouth.

i. Neck cysts

Symptoms
- Swelling and pain.

Signs
- Soft, tender swelling.
- Variable in size may be up to 10 cm in diameter.
- Superficial.
- Anterior to sternocleidomastoid near to the angle of the mandible.

Diagnostic tests
- Ultrasound valuable as is fluid filled.
- Biopsy: > 90% lined with stratified squamous epithelium. The walls contain lymphoid tisssue.

ii. Parotid cysts
- Cysts also occur in the parotid gland.
- Male:female ratio, 3:1.
- Important to differentiate from neoplasms, particularly the mucoepidermoid carcinoma.
- Unilateral or bilateral.

NB. Multiple lympho-epithelial cysts of the parotid, together with cervical lymphadenopathy are also seen in patients *infected with HIV* who present with *painless enlargement* of the parotid glands.

Diagnostic tests
- Computed tomographic (CT) scanning: shows multiple parotid cysts.
- Magnetic resonance imaging (MRI): multiple cysts.
- Fine needle aspiration: lymphocytes and epithelial cells.
- Biopsy: Multilocular cysts lined with epithelium surrounded by lymphoid tissue.

iii. Floor of the mouth and the tongue
- Generally symptomless.
- Non-ulcerated, freely movable masses.
- Usually on the lateral border in the case of the tongue.

Diagnostic tests
Radiography: no change shows.
Biopsy: epithelium surrounded by lymphoid tissue.
- Differential diagnosis includes mucoceles, lipomas or fibromas.

3. Thyroglossal duct cyst
- Develop from remnants of the thyroglossal duct.
- Equal sex distribution.
- Seen in all age groups but 30% reported in children less than 10 years old.

Symptoms
- May be a tender intraoral swelling.
- Can cause difficulty swallowing.

Signs
- Commonly located in the area of the hyoid bone.
- Intraorally appear either on the floor of the mouth or at the foramen caecum at the base of the tongue.
- Soft swelling, may be fluctuant.
- Rises when patient protrudes the tongue or swallows.
- Some have associated fistulae.
- Cases of squamous cell carcinoma developing in thyroglossal duct cysts have been reported.

Diagnostic tests
Biopsy: epithelially lined tract with thyroid tissue in the wall.

4. *Anterior median lingual cyst (intralingual cyst of foregut origin)*

Aetiology
Thought to be derived from inclusion of primitive foregut tissue during embryological development.

- Very rare.
- Present at birth.
- A cystic lesion on the anterior two-thirds of the tongue.
- Fluctuant.

5. *Oral cysts with gastric or intestinal epithelium (oral alimentary tract cyst)*

Aetiology
The origin of the aberrant tissue is unknown.

- Rare.
- Most cases reported in children.
- Present on tongue, floor of mouth, neck, and submandibular salivary gland.
- Male to female ratio 3:1.

Biopsy: cysts contain gastric and intestinal mucosa.

6. *Cystic hygroma*
- A developmental abnormality resulting in dilatation of lymph channels.
- Often present at birth and frequently involves the head and neck region.
- The face can be affected but not the mouth.
- Presents as a painless swelling which transilluminates.
- Skin over swelling may be blue.

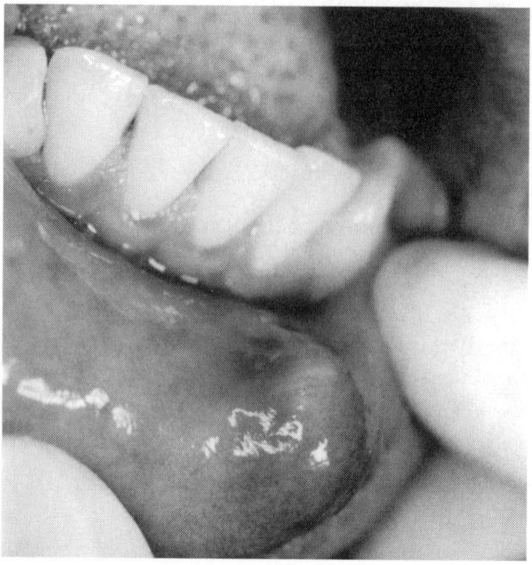

Figure 9.6 Mucocele on lower lip.

7, 8. Nasopharyngeal cysts and thymic cysts

- Both rare.
- Nasopharyngeal cysts may be midline or lateral.
- Thymic cysts arise from persistent thymic tissue.
- Seen between the angle of the mandible and the midline of the upper neck to the sternal notch.

9. Cysts of the salivary glands

Mucoceles (Fig. 9.6)

Symptoms

- Painless swellings usually of the lower lip.
- Caused by trauma to the minor salivary glands or their ducts.

Signs

- Soft, blue, fluctuant swellings on lower lip.

Diagnostic tests

Biopsy:

- May be extravasation cysts, where mucus has extravasated into the surrounding connective tissue and there is no epithelial lining, or

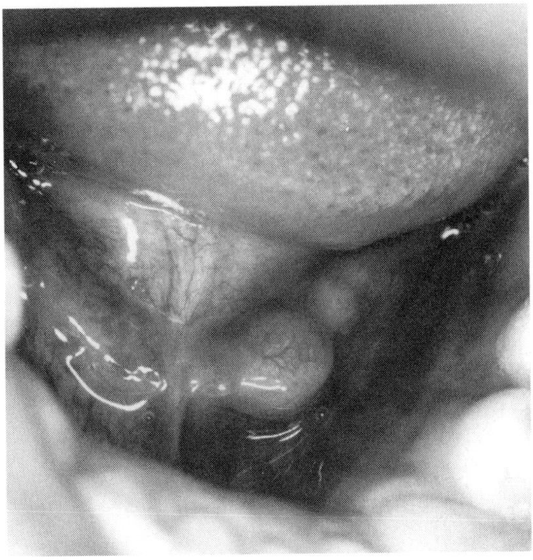

Figure 9.7 Ranula.

- Mucus retention cysts, which occur far less frequently and do have an epithelial lining.
- Retention cysts may be more frequent in older patients.

Differential diagnosis includes fibro-epithelial polyps and minor salivary gland tumours.

Ranula (Fig 9.7)
- A type of mucocele.
- Looks like a 'frog's belly'. Hence the name ranula (little frog).

Symptoms
- Slow-growing and painless swelling of floor of mouth.

Signs
- A unilateral swelling on the floor of the mouth.
- Often blue in colour and translucent.
- The majority have no epithelial lining.
- Can be further divided into superficial and plunging varieties.
- Plunging ranulae are thought to be mucus extravasation cysts derived from the sublingual gland.
- They herniate through the mylohyoid muscle and spread into the neck.

Diagnostic tests
- Biopsy: confirms the diagnosis.

Polycystic (dysgenetic) disease of the parotid glands
- Probably of developmental origin.
- Very rare, only a few cases ever recorded.
- Has occurred only in females.

Symptoms
- Bilateral, parotid swellings.
- Fluctuant and non tender.

Diagnostic tests
Sialography confirms cystic change within the parenchyma of the glands.

10. Parasitic cysts

Hydatid cysts
- Caused by the dog tapeworm *Echinococcus granulosus*.
- May occur as a painless swelling on the tongue.
- Also reported cases of lesions in the cheek and infratemporal fossa.
- Biopsy: confirms the diagnosis.

Further reading

Kramer, I.R.H., Pindborg, J.J. and Shear, M. (1992) *Histological Typing of Odontogenic Tumours*, 2nd edn. Berlin: Springer-Verlag.
Shear, M. (1992) *Cysts of the Oral Regions*, 3rd edn. Oxford: Wright.

10

Ulcers

Summary

Definition

History

Examination

Differential diagnosis

1. Traumatic
Sharp edge of a fractured tooth, overextended denture
Thermal and chemical burns
Iatrogenic — including radiotherapy/chemotherapy

2. Infective
Bacterial (TB, ANUG, syphilis)
Viral (herpes simplex, herpes zoster, cytomegalovirus, coxsackie, HIV, HHV8, i.e. human herpesvirus 8)
Fungal (histoplasmosis, mucormycosis, aspergillosis, cryptococcosis, blastomycosis and candidiasis—very rare)

3. Neoplastic
Squamous cell carcinoma
Kaposi's sarcoma (HHV8 infection)
Non-Hodgkin's lymphoma
Malignant melanoma
Malignant salivary gland tumours

4. Systemic
Mucous membrane pemphigoid
Pemphigus
Erythema multiforme
Lichen planus
Systemic lupus erythematosus (see Chapter 13)
Gastrointestinal disorders (Crohn's disease, ulcerative colitis) (see Chapter 13)
Haematological disorders (anaemias, neutropenias, leukaemia, immunosuppression, e.g. AIDS) (see Chapter 13)

5. Miscellaneous
Behçet's syndrome
Necrotizing sialometaplasia
Recurrent aphthous stomatitis
Drug-induced, e.g. gold injections for rheumatoid arthritis (lichenoid reaction) (see Chapter 12)

Definition

An ulcer is a pathological condition in which there is a breakdown of epithelial tissue.

There is full thickness loss of surface epithelium, with exposure of the underlying connective tissue.

In the mouth, ulcers are usually painful, except most importantly malignant oral tumours, which may be initially painless. Biopsy is therefore essential to establish the diagnosis of any ulcer that does not respond to treatment or persists for more than two to three weeks.

History

A detailed history is an essential component of the diagnosis.

The age of the patient is important. (Viral infections, recurrent aphthae are more common in children and adolescents. Erosive lichen planus, mucous membrane pemphigoid and squamous cell carcinoma, for example, affect middle-aged to elderly patients.)

Ask your patient:

How long have you had the ulcer(s)?

- A painless ulcer which has been present in an elderly patient for several weeks suggests carcinoma.

How many are there?

- Multiple suggests viral. If multiple and recurrent — aphthous ulceration.

Where is the ulcer located?

- ANUG affects the interdental papillae at first. Aphthous ulcers rarely affect the gingival margins.

Is it painful?

- Most ulcers are painful.
- However, early stages of oral carcinoma are often painless.

Do you know of anything that may have caused the ulcer, e.g. trauma, eating hot or heavily spiced food?

Have you ever had any ulcers before?

- Recurrent vesicles/ulcers on the lips and other mucocutaneous junctions likely to be herpes simplex.
- Recurrent intraoral ulcers — aphthae.

If yes, when? How many? How often? How long do they last?

Are there any associated problems, e.g. pain, bleeding, halitosis?

Is it getting bigger, smaller or staying the same size? (Smaller suggests healing. Becoming larger and painful could indicate a more serious aetiology.)

Do you get tingling or itching before the ulcers appear?
- Indicates possible viral aetiology, e.g. herpes simplex/zoster, or aphthae.

Do the ulcers start as blisters?
- Pemphigus, mucous membrane pemphigoid.

Do you get ulcers at other body sites, e.g. skin, eyes, genital regions?
- Behçet's syndrome, erythema multiforme.

Do you smoke? If so, how many cigarettes per day and for how long?
- Increased risk of oral cancer in heavy smokers and alcohol drinkers.

Do you drink alcohol? If yes, how many units per week? (A glass of wine/measure of spirits/half pint of beer equals 1 unit. Greater than 21 units for a man and 14 for a woman exceeds the government's recommended safe level of consumption of alcohol.)
Do you chew tobacco? If so, how much and how often.
- Increased risk of oral squamous cell carcinoma.

Do you chew betel quid? If so, how often?
- Leads to submucous fibrosis (a premalignant condition).

A comprehensive past medical history is also required (include medications and serious skin, gastrointestinal and haematological illnesses).

Examination of an ulcer

Use a systematic approach.

Site May give a clue to the cause.
- e.g. adjacent to a sharp tooth edge — trauma; interdental papilla — ANUG.

Posterior part of the mouth — coxsackie virus, e.g. herpangina.
- *Record* site in notes, draw diagram or take photographs.
- *Number* of ulcers (record number in notes).
- *Size* — measure in mm and draw in notes. Multiple ulcers suggests viral infection, e.g. coxsackie, herpes; or recurrent aphthae.
- *Shape* — e.g. round or crescentic (e.g. traumatic ulcers). Irregular and coalescing (e.g. viral such as CMV — irregular; or herpes — coalescing). Angular or stellate (TB). Punched out (tertiary syphilis).

- *Floor* — note the colour, the presence of a slough, scab, fungating, granulation or bleeding.
- *Base* — indurated, fixed to deeper structures. Induration and fixation suggest malignancy.
- *Edge* — raised, rolled and everted (malignant ulcers). Undermined/overhanging (tuberculous ulcers). Punched out (tertiary syphilitic ulcers). Rolled and pearly (rodent ulcers, extraoral on the face).

Associated problems

Secondary infection

- N.B. Take patient's temperature.

Pain

- Inflammatory and infective ulcers are painful.
- Malignant ulcers are often painless in the early stages.

Reactive lymphadenopathy

- Inhibits eating and speech.

Important — children may become dehydrated.

1. Traumatic ulcers

- Site may be adjacent to a carious or fractured tooth, the periphery of a denture or an orthodontic appliance.
- Patients will often recall the traumatic event.
- Traumatic ulcers are usually single, of variable size and round or crescentic in shape.
- The floor is yellow, the margins red and there is no induration.
- Traumatic ulcers should heal within a few days, after removal of the cause.

If an ulcer persists for more than two/three weeks without any evidence of healing, a biopsy must be taken to rule out other more sinister causes, e.g. squamous cell carcinoma.

Other possible causes of traumatic ulceration include :
- Accidental or deliberate biting.
- Thermal burns of the tongue and palate from hot foods, e.g. hot cheese dishes or pizza.

- Ingestion of caustic liquids.
- Placing an aspirin in the buccal sulcus for relief of toothache causes localized sloughing and superficial erosion.
- Iatrogenic — use of caustic dental medicaments, e.g. trichloracetic acid, beechwood creosote, eugenol and chromic acid.
  Ulcers from contact with hot dental instruments.
  Ulcers from removal of cotton wool rolls in the buccal sulcus.
  Following radiotherapy and chemotherapy the oral mucosa readily ulcerates after minimal trauma.

2. Infective ulcers

Bacterial

i. Tuberculosis (see also page 147)

- *Rare*. Occurs in patients with untreated, open pulmonary tuberculosis, who are coughing up infected sputum.

Symptoms
Progressive pain which significantly interferes with nutrition.

Oral signs

- Site — typically the dorsum of the tongue. The lips and palate are less often affected.
- Shape — angular or stellate.
- Floor — pale in colour with a thick mucus-like material in the base of the ulcer.
- Edge — irregular with an undermined border.

Associated systemic problems

- Chronic cough, weight loss, fever, night sweats and haemoptysis.

Diagnostic tests (see page 147)

Treatment

- No specific treatment for oral lesions is required. They heal with systemic treatment for the pulmonary infection.

ii. Acute necrotising ulcerative gingivitis (see page 92)

iii. Syphilis (see also page 148)
This is a notifiable disease and referral to a genito-urinary clinic is essential in all suspected cases.

Primary syphilis

- The classic lesion of primary syphilis is the chancre, usually on the genitalia. Rarely seen in or around the oral cavity.

Symptoms

- Painless unless secondarily infected.

Signs

- Site — the lip, tip of tongue, rarely other sites in the oral cavity.
- Size — variable from 5 mm to several centimetres in diameter.
- Shape — round.
- Edge — raised and indurated.
- Number of ulcers — usually single.

Associated problems

- Regional lymph nodes are enlarged, rubbery and discrete.
- The appearance of the ulcer, with its indurated edges, resembles a squamous cell carcinoma.
- Chancres heal spontaneously without scarring.
- Highly infectious.

Secondary syphilis

- Appears 3–12 weeks after the primary lesion (in untreated patients) as a papular or macular skin rash.
- Oral lesions are rarely seen without the rash appearing.

Symptoms

- The ulcers are painless.

Signs

- Site — palate, tonsils, lateral borders of the tongue and lips.
- Shape — flat, irregular ulcers covered by a grey membrane (snail track ulcers) when linear. They coalesce to form rounded areas known as mucous patches.

Associated problems

- Fever and malaise.
- Generalized lymphadenopathy
- Skin rash on palms.
- Highly infective.
- Serology positive at the secondary stage.

Tertiary syphilis

- Now very rarely seen.

- Occurs in *untreated cases* many years later.
- The lesion of the tertiary stage is the gumma, a destructive granulomatous process.

Symptoms
- Painless.

Signs
- Site — usually the palate, also tonsils and tongue.
- Size — variable from a few millimetres to several centimetres in diameter.
- Shape — round, punched-out appearance.
- Floor — depressed, with a pale (wash leather) appearance.
- Edge — punched-out.

Associated problems
- Syphilitic leukoplakia on the dorsum of the tongue. Very rare. High risk of malignant change.
- Neurosyphilis or involvement of the cardiovascular system affects 20% of patients. This may cause aortitis and subsequent thoracic aortic aneurysm, tabes dorsalis, dementia and general paresis of the insane.

Diagnostic tests (see page 149)

Viral infections

i. Primary herpetic gingivostomatitis
- Caused by herpes simplex virus type 1 (HSV 1) in most cases.
- Type 2 (HSV 2) of the oral cavity can occur (< 5% of cases).
- A DNA virus transmitted by saliva and direct contact.
- More common in children but also may occur in young adults.
- Primary infection is often subclinical.
- 90% of adults have antibodies to HSV 1 before 30 years of age and are carrying the virus in a latent form
- Remains dormant after infection in sensory ganglia.
- Subsequent reactivation of latent virus can occur and causes herpes labialis, the 'cold sore'.
- Initial infection may cause minimal symptoms or present as primary herpetic gingivostomatitis.

Symptoms
- Multiple oral ulcers causing painful gums, tongue and sore throat.

- Lips may be crusted with blood.
- Swallowing, eating, talking are all very painful.
- The patient feels unwell and will have a raised temperature.
- Nausea, vomiting and headache can be present.

Signs

- All parts of the mouth may be affected particularly the lips, gingivae, hard palate and tongue.
- Initially develop as vesicles which rupture.
- Gingivae are swollen and oedematous.
- Ulcers are multiple and coalesce.
- Shape — round and shallow.
- Size — 2–3 mm in diameter.
- Floor — yellow or grey.
- Edge — red, inflamed margins to ulcers.
- Occasional skin rashes.
- Temperature is raised and regional lymph nodes are enlarged and tender.
- Dehydration in children.

Recurrent infection

- Reactivation gives rise to herpes labialis, the 'cold sore' at mucocutaneous junctions.
- The lips are most frequently affected.

Predisposing factors include:

- Sunlight and cold.
- Psychological stress.
- Menstruation and occasionally pregnancy.
- Trauma.
- Systemic illness, e.g. common cold, influenza.
- Immune suppression, e.g. HIV.
- The virus is present in both the cold sores and saliva. Before the routine use of gloves, herpes simplex was occasionally transmitted to dental staff and caused herpetic whitlows. These are very painful infections of the fingers, especially the nail beds.

Symptoms

- Itching, or tingling sensation during the prodromal phase.
- Crops of vesicles appear after 24 hours on the lips.
- Rarely painful oral ulcers occur on the palate (multiple and coalescent).
- The buccal mucosa may also be affected.
- Slight tiredness and malaise common.

Signs

- Site — multiple small coalescing vesicles at the junction of the vermilion border and the skin of the lip. Can also affect the side of the nose.
- Vesicles become crusted and heal without scarring
- Regional lymph nodes may be tender and enlarged.
- Intraorally multiple, small, 1–2 mm ulcers which also coalesce may rarely be present. Buccal mucosa and the palate are affected.
- Application of 5% aciclovir cream during the prodromal phase lessens the clinical course.

ii. Herpes zoster (see pages 103–105)

N.B. There is an increased susceptibility to severe and potentially fatal herpes zoster infections in patients with HIV, Hodgkin's disease, leukaemia and those taking immunosuppressant drugs, including steroids, following organ transplantation.

iii. Cytomegalovirus

- The cause of the rare salivary gland swelling, cytomegalic inclusion disease in immunocompromised patients and babies.
- Can also cause oral ulceration in the immunocompromised patient, e.g. those receiving immunosuppressive drugs following organ transplantation or with HIV infection.
- Can be part of a widespread infection in patients with AIDS/HIV who develop retinitis, pneumonitis and meningoencephalitis.

Symptoms

- A painful, persistent, single ulcer.
- Painful when eating, swallowing and talking.

Signs

- Site — seen on the dorsum of tongue and also the buccal mucosa.
- Shape — elliptical or stellate.
- Floor — pale, grey colour.
- Size — may be large, greater than 1 cm.
- Edges — are irregular and undermined.

iv. Coxsackie virus

- Causes herpangina and hand, foot and mouth disease usually in children.
- May produce minor epidemics in schools or other institutions.
- Symptoms generally mild.

Herpangina

Symptoms
- Sore throat, feverish, feel unwell.

Signs
- Raised temperature and lymphadenopathy.
- Rarely salivary gland enlargement occurs as in mumps. Definitive diagnosis when there is doubt requires specialist laboratory support.
- Site — multiple vesicles and ulcers on the soft palate and tonsillar region.
- Size — small 1–2 mm.
- Shape — round and shallow.
- Surrounding mucosa red and inflamed.

Hand, foot and mouth disease
A mild illness with minimal systemic symptoms. There is a vesicular rash on the hands and feet in addition to the oral ulceration.

Symptoms
- Sore, tender, oral mucosa.
- Eating and swallowing increases the discomfort.
- Rash on hands and feet.

Signs
- Site — multiple ulcers on the tongue, buccal mucosa and the hard palate. The gingiva are *not* affected.
- Size — small, 1–2 mm, round and shallow.
- Surrounding mucosa red and inflamed.
- Macular and vesicular lesions on the hands and feet. Legs and arms may also be affected.

v. HIV (see also page 152)
Oral ulceration is seen in patients with AIDS and HIV (2% in one study) but the ulcers are not exclusive to patients infected with HIV.
- Ulcerative, oral lesions described in HIV are seen in the following:

Table 10.1 Ulcerative oral lesions described in HIV

Group 1 lesions strongly associated with HIV infection
• Necrotizing ulcerative gingivitis.
• Necrotizing ulcerative periodontitis.
• Kaposi's sarcoma.
• Non-Hodgkin's lymphoma.
Group 2 lesions (less commonly associated with HIV)
• Mycobacterium tuberculosis
• Necrotizing ulcerative stomatitis.
Viral infections
• Herpes simplex virus.
• Varicella zoster virus.
• *Ulceration not otherwise specified*
Group 3 lesions (seen in HIV infection)
• Erythema multiforme — due to a drug reaction.
Fungal infections
• Cryptococcosis.
• Histoplasmosis.
• Mucormycosis.
• Aspergillosis.
Recurrent aphthous stomatitis
Viral infection
• Cytomegalovirus.

Fungal infections

The 'deep mycoses' are rare but important conditions

- Rarely seen in UK residents.
- Are fungal organisms that can infect the oral cavity and head and neck region in patients who are resident in endemic regions or who are immunocompromised, e.g. patients with leukaemia or HIV disease.

i. Histoplasmosis

- Typically caused by *Histoplasma capsulatum*.
- Not naturally present in the UK.
- Endemic in certain parts of the world, e.g. Mississippi river valley region in the USA, Africa, South-East Asia and Australia.
- Seen in patients who are immunocompromised or from the endemic areas.

Symptoms
- Multiple, painful ulcers which may present anywhere in the mouth.
- Fever and cough.

Signs
- Site — lips, tongue, palate, gingiva and buccal mucosa can all be affected.
- Shape — may be nodular or vegetative lesions, or round ulcers.
- Floor — indurated and covered with a grey membrane.
- Resembles neoplastic change seen in squamous cell carcinoma.
- Enlarged regional lymph nodes may be present.

Diagnosis — by culture and histopathological examination of a biopsy specimen.

ii. Mucormycosis
- Occurs in the immunosuppressed.
- Also seen in severe, poorly controlled diabetic patients.
- Usually begins as a sinus infection which spreads intraorally.

Symptoms
- When the maxillary sinus is involved, facial pain, nasal discharge which may be blood stained and oral ulceration can occur.
- Can spread to the orbit, resulting in blindness, coma and death.
- May mimic dental pain.

Signs
- Site — the palate is usually involved. Also reported on gingiva, lip and alveolus.
- Size — may be large, greater than 1 cm.
- Floor — black slough.

Diagnosis — by culture and biopsy.

iii. Aspergillosis
- Also causes opportunistic infections in immunocompromised and poorly controlled diabetic patients.

Symptoms and signs — as for mucormycosis.

Diagnosis — by culture and biopsy.

iv. Cryptococcosis

- Also an opportunist infection in immunocompromised patients, e.g. AIDS, leukaemia and lymphoma.
- The lungs, skin and meninges as well as the oral cavity may be affected.

Symptoms

- Painful single or multiple ulcers.

Signs

- Appearance — non-specific.
- Site — usually the palate.
- Floor — necrotic.
- Size — may be large, several centimetres in diameter.
- Number — usually single.

Diagnosis — biopsy and culture.

v. Blastomycosis

- Very rare in the UK.
- As with histoplasmosis, endemic in the USA and South America.
- Much more common in men.
- Liver, lung and skin lesions seen.
- Oral lesions may begin as circumscribed nodules.

Symptoms

- Multiple mouth ulcers.
- Pustules discharging onto the face. Resembles actinomycosis.
- Weight loss, fever, cough (with pulmonary involvement) and swollen lymph glands.

Signs

- Pyrexia.
- Regional lymph nodes enlarged.
- Multiple small ulcers with rolled and indurated edges, resembling squamous cell carcinoma.

Diagnosis — biopsy and culture.

3. Neoplastic ulcers

Malignant

Oral tumours may present as mouth ulcers or exophytic growths.

i. Squamous cell carcinoma

- The most common oral malignancy (95% of cases).
- Accounts for 2–3% of all malignant tumours in the UK and the USA.
- Peak incidence between 55 and 75 years (> 70% of cases).
- More common in males.
- 2000 new cases in the UK each year.
- Increasing incidence in the UK.

Aetiological factors

- Tobacco and alcohol consumption.
- Chewing betel quid.
- Sunlight (skin and lip cancer).

Possible predisposing factors

- Oral epithelial dysplasia.
- Lichen planus.
- Chronic hyperplastic candidiasis.
- Haematinic deficiency.
- Syphilitic leukoplakia (very rare).

Symptoms

- Often initially painless, may be overlooked or ignored by patients.
- Becomes painful when infected or when the tumour invades neural tissue.
- Swollen non-tender glands in the neck.
- Swallowing, eating and talking become dificult and painful with advanced disease.
- Loosening of the teeth in carcinoma of the gingiva, or through spread to bone.

Signs

- Site — tongue, floor of mouth, buccal mucosa, alveolar ridge (account for > 60% of all oral cancer).
- Shape — round, crescentic or irregular.
- Edge — raised, rolled and everted.
- Floor — granular and ragged, may bleed easily.
- Base — indurated and fixed to deeper tissues.

Lymphatic spread

- Spreads to the regional lymph nodes. 30% of patients have lymph node involvement at presentation.
- Enlarged nodes become firm or hard, are non-tender and may be fixed to adjacent tissue.

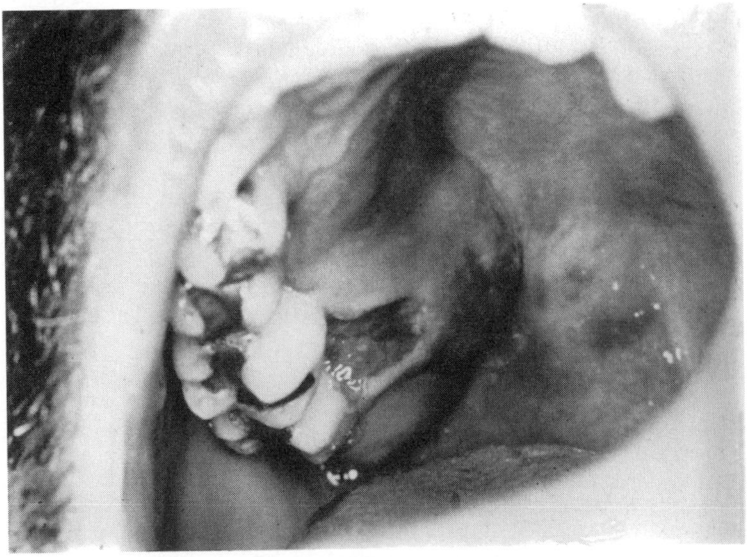

Figure 10.1 Kaposi's sarcoma with palatal ulceration.

- Lymphadenopathy may be the initial clinical presentation of carcinoma of the tongue.

Diagnostic tests
- Biopsy and histopathological examination, plain radiology, computerized tomography (CT), magnetic resonance imaging (MRI), bone scintigraphy and ultrasound (rarely).

ii. Kaposi's sarcoma (Fig. 10.1)
- An AIDS defining illness in HIV-positive patients.
- Disseminated Kaposi's sarcoma is a frequent cause of death in AIDS.
- A tumour of microvascular endothelial tissue now known to be caused by human herpes virus 8 (HHV 8).

Symptoms
- Early changes present as *painless*, flat areas of pigmentation of the mucosa or the gingiva.
- As lesions increase in size they become raised.
- Large lesions can make eating and talking uncomfortable.
- May eventually ulcerate, causing constant pain.

Signs

- Typically single or multiple blue/red/purple, macules/papules/nodules or ulcers.
- *Advanced* lesions may show a central area of ulceration.
- Site — the most common site is the palate opposite the upper molar teeth.
- Shape — begin as flat, blue/red/purple macules. As lesions increase in size they become nodular and raised, similar in clinical appearance to haemangiomas or ecchymoses.
- Number — single or multiple lesions that eventually coalesce.
- Size — variable from a few millimetres to several centimetres.
- Floor of ulcer — grey, necrotic, may bleed.
- Edges — red with no induration.

Diagnosis

- Biopsy and histopathological examination.

HIV antibody test is appropriate in patients whose status is unknown but only after appropriate counselling and with the patient's full informed consent. Referral to a specialist genito-urinary medicine clinic is necessary when considering testing.

Occasionally oral Kaposi's sarcoma can occur in other (non-HIV related) immunosuppressive states, e.g. long-term cyclosporin therapy.

iii. Non-Hodgkin's lymphoma

- A malignant tumour of lymphoid tissue which may present as oral ulceration.
- Also an AIDS defining illness in HIV-positive patients. May be either of B cell or T cell origin.

Symptoms

- Painless enlargement of the cervical lymph nodes may be the initial complaint.
- Can cause painful intraoral ulceration and facial swelling.
- Limited jaw opening.

Signs

- Site — gingiva, palate, buccal mucosa and pharynx.
- Shape — round or irregular.
- Floor — yellow, may bleed due to trauma.
- Margins — red and inflamed.
- Cervical lymphadenopathy.
- Trismus, when facial and masticatory muscles are involved.

- Facial swelling when the buccal sulcus is affected.
- Occasionally there can be extensive alveolar bone destruction, resulting in tooth mobility or loss and oroantral communications.

Diagnostic tests
- Biopsy and histopathological examination. Usually additional immunohistochemical analyses are required.
- Radiology. Can cause bone loss in adjacent teeth.

iv. Malignant melanoma
- Rare in the mouth. Has a very poor prognosis.
- Most patients are 30+ years of age.
- Twice as common in males.

Symptoms
- An area of mucosal pigmentation which is increasing in size.
- The lesion may bleed and ulcerate.

Signs
- Site — hard palate and maxillary gingiva/alveolar ridge (80% of cases).
- Size — variable, a few millimetres in diameter or may be large >1 cm
- Shape — irregular outline. Black, brown or red in colour.
- Floor — bleeds in later stages.

Associated problems — metastasize early.

- Any hyperpigmented, melanotic oral lesion with irregular margins or a history of growth, should be treated with the utmost suspicion and early biopsy.
- Poor prognosis, 5 year survival rate approximately 5%.

v. Malignant salivary gland tumours (see also page 253)
- May present as an ulcerated swelling in the oral cavity, typically the palate.

Symptoms
- Begins as a painless swelling in the palate.
- Painful when ulcerated

Signs
- Site — usually the hard palate. Can also occur on the lips and buccal mucosa.
- Size variable. Can extend to several centimetres.

Diagnostic tests

- Biopsy and histopathological examination, computerized tomography (CT) scanning, magnetic resonance imaging (MRI).

4. Systemic ulcers

i. Mucous membrane pemphigoid

- An autoimmune disease, causing loss of epithelial attachment to the underlying connective tissue.
- A chronic condition occurring mainly in patients over 50 years of age.
- Four times more common in women.
- Affects the eyes, and skin as well as the oral mucosa.
- The oesophagus, larynx and trachea may also be involved.
- Eye involvement is particularly serious as conjunctival scarring can lead to loss of vision.

Symptoms

- Painful, blood-filled blisters (vesicles and bullae).
- These rupture to form ulcers and erosions on mucosal surfaces.
- The gingiva are particularly affected, giving rise to sore and painful gums (desquamative gingivitis).

Signs

- Site — soft palate frequently affected and gingivae. Erosions may also be seen on the buccal mucosa.
- Size — blood-filled, bullae/vesicles may be several centimetres in diameter.
- Shape — round, although both the ulcers and erosions can be irregular.
- Edge — ruptured bullae have well-defined margins.
- Floor — ruptured bullae have an inflamed base.

Associated problems

- Rarely, intraoral lesions may heal with scarring.
- Fibrosis of the oesophagus, larynx and trachea can lead to strictures, resulting in difficulty in swallowing or breathing.
- Patients must be referred for an ophthalmology examination as up to 75% of patients can have conjunctival involvement with subsequent scarring and possible loss of vision.

Diagnosis

- Biopsy and immunofluorescent microscopy (direct and

indirect). Circulating autoantibodies may be present in 5% of patients. Fresh, unfixed specimens are required for direct immunofluorescence.

ii. Pemphigus

- An autoimmune disease of skin and mucous membrane with *intra*epithelial vesicles or bullae.
- Fatal if untreated, although therapy can itself be hazardous.
- More common in women 40–60 years of age.
- 50% of cases initially present with oral lesions.
- Lesions begin as vesicles or bullae. These are fragile and easily traumatized in the mouth.

Symptoms

- Patients present with shallow, painful oral ulcers, which bleed easily.
- Eating, talking and swallowing are painful.
- Large fluid-filled blisters are present on the skin.

Signs

- Vesicles and bullae may be several centimetres in diameter covering large areas of the skin surface. The lesions contain a clear fluid initially which soon becomes blood stained or purulent.

Intraorally

- Site — buccal mucosa, palate, gingiva, i.e. sites which are easily traumatized.
- Number — multiple.
- Size — variable from a few millimetres to several centimetres.
- Shape — irregular, with a ragged border.
- Floor — the ulcers are shallow, with a denuded base and are often covered with a white or bloodstained exudate.
- When the lips are affected, they become bloodstained and crusted.
- The epithelium peels away and the edges continue to extend until large areas of the oral mucosa are involved.

Complications.

- Bacterial septicaemia with *Staphylococcus aureus*.
- Extensive skin involvement leads to loss of fluids and electrolytes.
- Potentially fatal, patients must be referred for specialist dermatological care.

Diagnostic tests
- Stroking the mucosa gently may produce a bulla or vesicles (Nikolsky's sign).
- Pressure on an intact bulla increases the size of the lesion.

Biopsy
- Shows acantholysis (loss of attachment of epithelial cells to each other).
- Direct and indirect immunofluorescent antibody tests demonstrate binding of IgG, IgM and C3 deposits in the intercellular substance of the epithelial tissue and a raised titre of IgG antibodies respectively.

iii. Erythema multiforme
- Sudden onset.
- Young adults predominantly affected.
- More common in males.
- Variable clinical appearance, hence the name 'multiforme'.
- May have recurrent episodes.
- When only the mouth is affected, can appear identical, clinically, to primary herpetic gingivostomatitis.
- A history of previous episodes or cold sores, eliminates primary herpes from the differential diagnosis.
- Can be a reaction to a precipitating or trigger agent, for example:
- Drugs — sulphonamides, trimethoprim, barbiturates, penicillin and nitrofurantoin.
- Infection — herpes simplex, mycoplasmal pneumonia.
- Other triggers include benign and malignant tumours, radiotherapy, Crohn's disease, sarcoidosis, histoplasmosis and infectious mononucleosis. In many patients no cause can be found, although underlying herpetic infection is likely.

Symptoms
- Painful, oral erosions and ulcers.
- Lesions widespread affecting large areas of the mouth.
- Lips crusted amd blood stained.
- Skin, ocular and genital lesions may be present.
- Fever, feel unwell (malaise), swollen glands.

Signs
Site:
- Multiple sites affected.
- Crusted and bleeding erosions present on lips.
- Intraoral ulcers and erosions on labial mucosa, tongue, gingiva, etc.

- Size — may be several centimetres in diameter.
- Shape — irregular outline with ill-defined margins.
- Edge — inflamed and erythematous.
- The patient is pyrexial, looks obviously ill and has tender, palpable, regional lymph nodes.
- Skin lesions known as target lesions, may occur on the hands and feet, in particular, and also on the face and neck.
- These appear as erythematous concentric rings.
- Can also affect the eyes and cause blindness, in rare cases.
- The patient's medical practitioner must be informed as severe cases require hospital admission to maintain an adequate intake of fluids.

iv. Erosive/ulcerative lichen planus

- Lichen planus is a disorder affecting the skin and the oral cavity.
- 70% of patients with skin lesions have oral involvement.
- But only *10%* of patients presenting with oral lesions have skin involvement.
- Affects 2% of the population.
- More common in women over 30 years of age.
- The aetiology is unknown.
- Six different subtypes of lichen planus have been described:
- Erosive (see below), reticular, papular and plaque-like (see Chapter 11), atrophic and bullous.
- *However, different types can be present in one patient at the same time and there may not be a clear distinction clinically.*

Symptoms of erosive lichen planus

- Erosions cause soreness and pain in the affected areas of the mouth, particularly on eating.
- Erosions appear suddenly but can taken weeks or months to heal.

Signs

- Shallow, irregular, erosions or ulcers.
- Site — the lesions are usually bilateral and affect the buccal mucosa, tongue, labial mucosa and gingiva. The palate and lingual gingiva are usually spared.
- Gingival atrophic lesions ('desquamative gingivitis') closely resemble those of mucous membrane pemphigoid.
- Size — millimetres to several centimetres in diameter.
- Floor — yellow with a layer of fibrin covering the base.
- Edge — may have sunken margins due to fibrosis and an erythematous border.
- Diagnosis — mucosal biopsy.

- Malignant transformation to squamous cell carcinoma is rare but has been suggested to be more likely in erosive than the other forms of lichen planus.

5. Miscellaneous ulcers

i. Behçet's syndrome

- Rare in the UK.
- Highest incidents of Behçet's syndrome in East Asia and East Mediterranean regions.
- More common in young men between the ages of 20 and 40.
- A multi-system disorder in which a common triad of features occur.
  1. Recurrent oral ulceration (of the aphthous type) described below in the section 'recurrent aphthous stomatitis.'
  2. Genital ulceration.
  3. Eye lesions.
- A multi-system disease with skin lesions, arthritis, thrombophlebitis and lesions of the nervous system, vascular system, gastrointestinal tract and pulmonary disease.
- In 1990 an international study group recommended the following diagnostic criteria for Behçet's syndrome:
  'Recurrent oral ulceration occurring at least three times in one 12-month period plus two of the following four manifestations.
  i. Recurrent genital ulceration.
  ii. Eye lesions including uveitis or retinal vasculitis.
  iii. Skin lesions including erythema nodosum, pseudo-folliculitis, papulo-pustular lesions or acneform nodules in a post-adolescent patient not receiving corticosteroids.
  iv. Positive pathergy (skin hyperreactivity, e.g. pustule formation after venepuncture).
- Oral ulceration may be of the minor or major recurrent aphthous type.
- Genital ulcers occur on the scrotum or penis in males and the vulva/labia in females.
- Eye lesions include uveitis, retinal infiltrates, conjunctivitis and retinal atrophy. May result in permanent scar damage or even blindness.
- Central nervous system involvement may involve cranial nerves or give rise to symptoms resembling multiple sclerosis.

ii. Necrotizing sialometaplasia

- Unknown aetiology — probably traumatic.
- Affects the minor salivary glands of the palate.

- More common in males 50–60 years of age.
- Now known to be an occasional feature of bulimia nervosa.

Symptoms
- A painful ulcer in the palate.

Signs
- Site — hard palate midway between the palatal raphe and gingival margin. Usually the molar region. Cases also reported on the lip and retromolar pad.
- Number — single.
- Size — may be large up to 2 cm in diameter.
- Shape — round with irregular margins.
- Base — often the palatal bone.
- Floor — yellow with necrotic debris.
- Edges — inverted or heaped up and indurated.

Important
- Resembles squamous cell carcinoma clinically.
- Histologically may also resemble squamous cell carcinoma and mucoepidermoid carcinoma.
- However, this condition is self-limiting and heals spontaneously in 2–3 months.

iii. Recurrent aphthous stomatitis
- A common cause of oral ulceration; recurrent aphthae affect up to 20% of the population.
- Similar incidence in males and females.
- The diagnosis is mainly by clinical examination and history, which is one of recurrent, painful oral ulcers in an otherwise well individual.
- Peak age of onset is the second decade of life.
- Associated factors include trauma, psychological stress, menstruation, and food allergies, e.g. chocolate and preservatives.
- Also associated with a deficiency of iron, folic acid and vitamin B_{12}.
- Aphthae may be more common in *non* tobacco smokers.

Three types of recurrent aphthae are described:
1. Minor aphthae — 80% of cases. Less than 1 cm in diameter. These heal without scarring.
2. Major aphthae — 10% of cases. Greater than 1 cm in diameter. Healing period lengthy (several weeks) and may be followed by scarring.

3. Herpetiform ulcers — 10% of cases. Multiple, up to 100 may be present at the same time. Small 1–2 mm.

Minor aphthous ulcers

Symptoms

- Painful recurrent mouth ulcers.
- Patients may experience a prodromal tingling sensation before the ulcers appear.
- As with any oral ulceration, eating, talking and swallowing will increase pain and discomfort.
- May have swollen and tender cervical lymph nodes.

Signs

- Site — buccal mucosa, labial mucosa, floor of mouth and occasionally the dorsum of the tongue. *Not present* on the keratinized gingivae or palatal mucosa.
- Number of ulcers — may be single or in crops of two to three. Occasionally multiple.
- Size — usually 2–5 mm in diameter.
- Shape — round or elliptical and shallow.
- Floor — yellow.
- Edges — inflamed with red margins.
- Lymphadenopathy if rare secondary infection occurs.

Major aphthae

Symptoms

- Large, recurrent painful ulcers.
- Eating, drinking and even swallowing their saliva can cause patients severe pain.
- Weight loss, due to pain when trying to eat.

Signs

- Site — principally, the posterior part of the mouth, including keratinized tissue.
- However, the whole of the oral cavity, including the non-keratinized mucosa of the soft palate and tonsillar areas, rarely affected by minor aphthae, can be the site of major apthous ulceration.
- Number of ulcers — single or multiple.
- Size — greater than 1 cm. May be as large as 5 cm.
- Shape — round or elliptical.
- Floor — yellow, grey.
- Edges — red and inflamed. May be heaped and raised.

- Base — remains soft and does not become indurated.
- Seen in patients with HIV infection (Group 2 lesion)

Herpetiform aphthae

Symptoms
- Multiple, painful, recurrent mouth ulcers.

Signs
- More common in females.
- Site — the tongue and floor of mouth and buccal mucosa
- Number of ulcers — multiple, as many as 100 at the same time. May coalesce and become confluent.
- Size — small 1–3 mm.
- Shape — irregular.
- Floor — grey.
- Edge — ill-defined.
- Widespread erythema of mucous membrane present.

Associated problems
Major aphthae heal slowly, can persist for up to 3 months and may scar.

Diagnostic tests
- As noted in the introduction, diagnosis is primarily from the history and examination.
- However, a haematological investigation is essential to identify any deficiency states. A full blood count, serum ferritin, vitamin B_{12} and red blood cell folate levels should therefore be requested.

Further reading

Cawson, R.A., Langdon, J.D. and Eveson, J.W. (1996) *Surgical Pathology of the Mouth and Jaws*, 1st edn. Oxford: Wright.
Eversole, L.R. (1996) *Oral Medicine: a Pocket Guide*, 1st edn. Philadelphia: Saunders.
Lamey, P.J. and Lewis, M.A.O. (1997) *A Clinical Guide to Oral Medicine*, 2nd edn. London: British Dental Association.

11

White patches

Summary

Introduction

History

Examination of a white patch

Differential diagnosis

Removable white patches

Differential diagnosis

- i. Milk curd (babies)
- ii. Epithelial or food debris
- iii. Leukoedema (removed by pressure on the mucosa)
- iv. Chemical trauma
- v. Pseudomembranous candidiasis/candidosis

Non-removable white patches

Differential diagnosis

A. Congenital

- i. White sponge naevus
- ii. Dyskeratosis follicularis

B. Acquired

Traumatic

1. Frictional keratosis
2. Smoker's keratosis
3. Submucous fibrosis

Infective

4. Candidal leukoplakia (chronic hyperplastic candidiasis/candidosis). See also pseudomembranous candidiasis
5. Syphilitic leukoplakia (very rare)
6. Oral hairy leukoplakia

Dermatological

7. Lichen planus and lichenoid drug reactions
8. Systemic lupus erythematosus
9. Discoid lupus erythematosus

Miscellaneous

10. Skin graft

continued

11. Vitamin A deficiency continued (see page 264)

Neoplasia and premalignant conditions

12. Leukoplakia
13. Speckled leukoplakia
14. Erythroplakia
15. Squamous cell carcinoma (verrucous carcinoma, see page 246).

Introduction

There are many conditions which present in the mouth as white patches. Some are considered to be premalignant or associated with malignancy. Whenever it is unclear as to the aetiology and diagnosis of a white patch, it is *essential* to obtain a definitive histological diagnosis. Taking a biopsy can be carried out in general dental practice. However, practitioners may prefer to refer patients to specialist units for diagnosis and treatment.

History

- A careful history is required and the following questions should be asked:
- How long have you had the white patch? (congenital or acquired).
- Has it ever been painful? If yes, consider chemical trauma, frictional trauma, chronic hyperplastic candidiasis (candidosis), atrophic or erosive lichen planus and discoid lupus erythematosus. Neoplastic and premalignant conditions are also painful when ulcerated or secondarily infected.
- Is there a history of trauma? (chemical, e.g. aspirin; frictional, e.g. sharp tooth or restoration).
- Do you smoke? Note daily amount and for how many years.
- Do you drink alcohol? Note weekly consumption in units and years of drinking (see also page 187).
- Do you chew betel or areca nuts?
- Do you chew tobacco?
- There is a significant association between the use of tobacco, alcohol and betel chewing and the incidence of leukoplakia/erythroplakia.
- A comprehensive medical history and family history should also be taken (see pages 7–9).

Examination of a white patch

- Clinical examination needs to be structured and the size and location of the lesion(s) recorded in the patient's notes. Draw the lesion(s) to scale or photograph. Note whether they are symmetrical.
- Careful examination of any dentures (for sharp edges or over extension) and orthodontic appliances is necessary, as is palpation to detect sharp teeth or fillings.
- Initially determine whether the patch is removable with a gauze or tongue spatula.
- Note any mucosal ulceration and erythema.
- Palpate for cervical lymph node enlargement.

N.B. When nodes are palpable this suggests that infection, inflammation or neoplasia may be present.

Removable white patches

If the white patch can be removed and there is *no* inflammation of the underlying mucosa, the differential diagnosis includes:

- i. Milk curd.
- ii. Epithelial or food debris.

Removable lesions with associated underlying pathology

- iii. Leukoedema.
- iv. Chemical trauma.
- v. Pseudomembranous candidiasis and other fungal disorders, e.g. mucormycosis.

Leukoedema

- Aetiology unknown.
- Not associated with epithelial dysplasia.
- And not a premalignant condition.
- Reported prevalence — varies widely.
- Significance uncertain.
- Reported more frequently in non-Caucasians possibly due to the greater colour contrast.

Symptoms

Asymptomatic.

Signs
- A filmy, white/grey coating on the buccal mucosa.
- Majority of cases bilateral.
- Can be 'removed' (by pressure on the cheek and stretching the mucosa).
- Represents a variant of normal oral mucosa.

If there is inflammation of the underlying mucosa consider:

Chemical trauma, e.g. history of placing aspirin in the buccal sulcus

Aspirin burn
- There will be a history of oral pain, e.g. toothache and placing an aspirin in the buccal sulcus.
- It causes a chemical burn of the mucosa resulting in a white patch (Fig. 11.1).
- Chemical burns can also occur with excessive use of tooth tinctures and clove oil.
- May occur accidentally during dental treatment, e.g. orthophosphoric acid etchant gel coming in contact with the gingiva or mucosa.

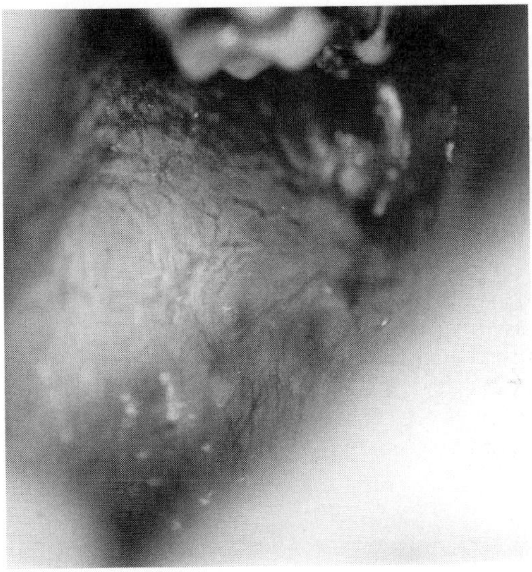

Figure 11.1 Aspirin burn on buccal mucosa.

Symptoms
- Mucosa painful in the area of burn.

Signs
- A white patch in the buccal mucosa, adjacent to the painful tooth.
- Can often be removed, exposing the inflamed, underlying mucosa.
- The source of the dental pain should be evident either clinically or radiographically.
- Sloughs in 1 or 2 days.
- Resolves without treatment or scarring.

Pseudomembranous candidiasis (candidosis)
See Chapter 8 page 154 for predisposing factors to candidal infection. Essential to establish the aetiology.

Symptoms
- May be asymptomatic.
- Can cause a sore, painful mouth.
- Discomfort on swallowing.
- Loss of taste.

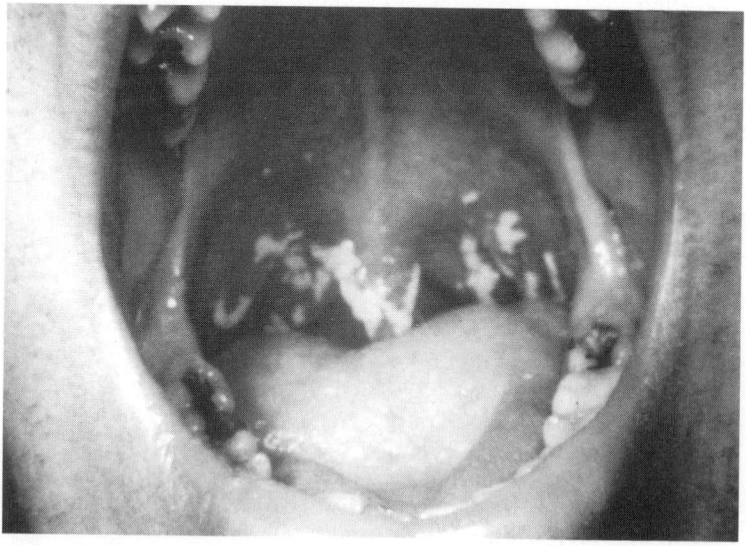

Figure 11.2 Pseudomembranous candidiasis.

Signs
- Creamy white/yellow patches which can be easily removed from the mucosa leaving behind an erythematous, sometimes bleeding, surface (Fig. 11.2).
- Can be extensive, covering the palate, tongue, buccal mucosa and throat.

Diagnostic tests
- Gram stain from a smear. Potassium hydroxide or periodic-acid Schiff may also be usd to demonstrate candidal hyphae.
- Culture from smear/swab to isolate the strain of candida.
- Quantification using a salivary candidal count or a 1 minute phosphate-buffered saline rinse.

Non-removable white patches

A. Congenital

i. White sponge naevus (familial white folded gingivostomatitis)
- An autosomal dominant congenital disorder.
- Equal gender distribution.
- May be present from birth but often first diagnosed during adolescence.
- Possible family history with others in the family similarly affected.

Symptoms
- Painless.

Signs
- Variable.
- However, large areas of the buccal mucosa and floor of mouth may be involved.
- Mucosa appears thickened and folded.
- Nasal mucosa may also be affected.
- A completely benign condition.
- No treatment required other than reassurance.
- Biopsy and histopathological examination confirms the diagnosis.

ii. Dyskeratosis follicularis (Darier's disease)
- An autosomal dominant, congenital disorder.
- Skin and mucosal lesions seen.
- Oral cavity affected in 50% of cases.

Symptoms
- Painless.

Signs
- Tiny, white, rough, papules.
- Cobblestone appearance of the mucosa.
- Occurs on the gingiva, tongue, palate and buccal mucosa.
- Other mucosal surfaces may also be involved, e.g. pharynx and larynx.
- Crusted skin lesions also seen.
- Red or grey/brown papules in skin folds, on neck, scalp and forehead.
- Diagnosis confirmed by biopsy.

B. Acquired

Traumatic

1. Frictional
- A detailed history will usually identify causes of traumatic injuries to the mucosa.
- Severe acute trauma will often cause ulceration.
- More chronic, low grade irritation gives rise to the white patch of frictional keratosis.
- This is confined to the traumatized area.

Causes

a. Cheek or lip biting
- The white patch may be unilateral or bilateral.
- Sometimes located at the level of the occlusal plane although in severe cases can affect all of the adjacent buccal mucosa.
- Also can affect the labial mucosa particularly the lower lip.
- Patients will usually admit to cheek biting if questioned specifically.

Relevant medical history: psychological stress and disorders, anxiety, self-inflicted injury, temporomandibular joint dysfunction.

b. Denture induced
- The white patch is related to the margins of an overextended or poorly fitting denture/orthodontic appliance.

c. Sharp tooth
- The white patch is adjacent to the sharp cusp or fractured tooth/restoration.

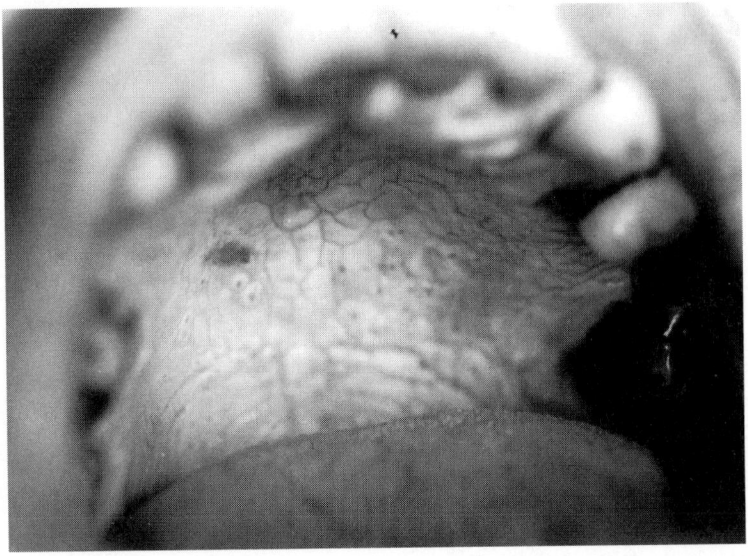

Figure 11.3 Smoker's keratosis.

- Adjacent tissue is usually normal in appearance.
- Majority are reversible, removal of the cause results in resolution.
- Essential to review after removing the cause in 2 to 3 weeks.
- Persistent white patches must be biopsied.

2. *Smoker's keratosis* (Fig. 11.3)
- A history of pipe smoking.
- May occur with cigarettes and cigars.

Symptoms
- Painless.

Signs
- Possible nicotine staining of teeth.
- White palatal mucosa with raised nodules projecting from the surface of the palate.
- The centre of the nodules are red. These are inflamed orifices of minor salivary glands.
- Resolution may occur if the patient stops smoking.

Essential for all persistent white patches
- All aetiological factors which cause trauma must be removed and patients reviewed within 2–3 weeks to ensure that the tissues have returned to a normal appearance.
- As noted above, any persistent or suspect white patches must always be biopsied to eliminate the possibility of malignant change.

3. Submucous fibrosis
- Typically affects certain Asian populations, e.g. Northern India and Bangladesh.
- Associated with an increased incidence of oral squamous cell carcinoma.
- Caused by chewing betel quid.
- Affected patients may have a genetic predisposition.

Symptoms
- Painless.
- May have a burning sensation with spicy foods.
- Marked limitation of opening.

Signs
- Patient of Indian or Bangladeshi origin.
- Variable trismus.
- The thick, fibrous tissue in the submucosal layer produces rigid bands in the buccal mucosa.
- Mucosa white and opaque.
- Cannot be indented with finger pressure.
- May be loss of the filiform papillae if the dorsum of the tongue is affected.

Infective

Candidiasis (candidosis)
4. Chronic hyperplastic candidiasis (candidal leukoplakia)
- Smoking strongly implicated as a co-factor in the aetiology of this condition.
- Potential for malignant change.

Symptoms
- Sore or painful commissures.

Signs
- Firmly adherent white areas at the commissures.
- Unilateral or bilateral.

- Can have a speckled or smooth appearance.
- May be ulcerated.
- Rarely resolves with long term use of systemic antifungals.
- Patients must be strongly advised to stop smoking.
- *Biopsy is required* to definitively confirm a diagnosis of candidal leukoplakia as the organisms are intraepithelial and not on the surface of the mucosa.
- Excisional biopsy may be required to eliminate the lesion if anti-fungal therapy fails.
- *Most important* this is considered to be premalignant.
- 7% over a 10 year period undergo malignant change.
- Long term follow up is essential.

5. Syphilitic leukoplakia
See also page 149.
- Very rare.
- White patches occur in the tertiary stage.

Symptoms
- Asymptomatic.

Signs
- Firmly adherent white patch on the dorsum of the tongue.
- High incidence of malignant change.

Diagnostic tests
- See page 149 for serological tests.

Viral

6. Oral hairy leukoplakia (Fig. 11.4)
Symptoms
- Usually symptom free.
- May be uncomfortable or interfere with speech if extensive and covers most of the dorsum of the tongue.
- Caused by the Epstein–Barr virus.
- Strongly associated with HIV disease but can occur in other immunocompromised states including corticosteroid therapy.

Signs
- A firmly adherent white patch, often forming hair-like strands, usually on the lateral border of the tongue.
- May occur on buccal mucosa and ventral/dorsal surfaces of the tongue also.

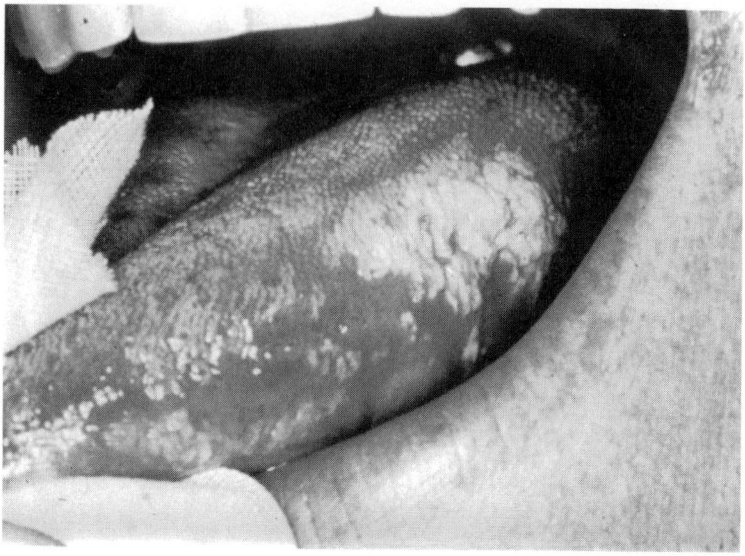

Figure 11.4 Oral hairy leukoplakia.

Diagnostic tests

- Biopsy and histopathological examination of tissue.
- Use of monoclonal antibodies to demonstrate Epstein–Barr virus in a biopsy of oral tissue or in epithelial cells obtained from scrapes of the affected mucosa.
- Most cases are symptom free and do not require treatment. Antiviral medications such as aciclovir will cause extensive lesions to regress but they are likely to recur once therapy has been stopped.

Dermatological

7. Lichen planus

- See also page 205.
- Affects 1–2% of the population.
- Majority of patients between 30 and 50 years of age.
- May also occur on the skin as well as the oral cavity.
- Skin lesions on the flexor surfaces of the wrist are papular and dusky pink in colour.
- Fine, lacy striations (Wickham's striae) are present on the papules.
- Different types of lichen planus have been described and may be present simultaneously.

Plaque-like
Reticular
Papular
Erosive see page 205
Atrophic
Bullous

Symptoms
- May be asymptomatic or sore, especially with hot and spicy foods.
- The atrophic and erosive varieties though, are often painful.

Signs
- Bilateral firmly adherent, white plaques usually on the buccal mucosa.
- May also affect the tongue, attached gingiva and lips.
- The palate and lingual surfaces of the gingivae are rarely involved.
- Patches are lacy and firmly adherent.
- Potential for malignant change.
- Biopsy required to confirm diagnosis in cases of doubt and to differentiate from lupus erythematosus.

Lichenoid drug reactions
- These white patches are identical clinically to lichen planus.
- They are caused by a mucosal reaction to certain drugs.

Signs and symptoms
- As for lichen planus.
- A positive drug history is essential in establishing a diagnosis.

Drugs known to cause lichenoid reactions include:
a. Some non steroidal anti-inflammatory drugs.
b. Antihypertensives, e.g. methyldopa, beta-adrenergic blockers.
c. Antimalarials.
d. Antimicrobials, e.g. tetracyclines and sulphonamides.
e. Lithium.
f. Phenothiazines.
g. Gold injections.
h. Dental amalgams, dental composites and glass ionomers implicated.
i. May appear in HIV disease, hepatitis C and as a complication of graft-versus-host disease.

As with all white patches it is essential to monitor patients with lichen planus and to re-biopsy any suspicious changes in the appearance of the mucosa. Patients should be strongly advised to stop smoking and reduce alcohol consumption.

8. Systemic lupus erythematosus
(See also page 281).
- 20% of patients with systemic lupus erythematosus at some stage of the disease have white patches on the oral mucosa that clinically resemble lichen planus.
- The antimalarials, e.g. hydroxychloroquine used to control systemic lupus erythematosus can also cause lichenoid reactions.
- Definitive diagnosis requires immunological investigations, as noted in Chapter 13, together with biopsy of the white patch and immunofluorescence.

9. Discoid lupus erythematosus
- Females mainly affected 2:l.
- 20–50% have oral changes.
- May be rash on face, hands and scalp.
- No significant systemic effects.

Symptoms
- Painful erosions of the lips and buccal mucosa.

Signs
- Firmly adherent, white patches on the lips and buccal mucosa.
- Fine white striae present with depressed central erythematous region.
- Often symmetrical, palatal lesions more common than in lichen planus.
- No induration present.
- As malignant transformation has been reported in these lesions, they must be monitored closely.

Diagnostic tests
- Biopsy and histopathological examination.

Miscellaneous

10. Skin graft
- Skin grafts are used to repair mucosal defects, e.g. following surgery for an oral malignancy.

- The patient's history confirms previous surgery and skin graft.

Symptoms
- Asymptomatic.

Signs
- White patch.
- May have hairs, depending on the location of the donor site.
- Sharply demarcated border where the white appearance of the skin graft joins the adjacent oral mucosa.

11. Vitamin A deficiency
(See page 264).

Neoplasia and premalignant conditions

12. Leukoplakia
- This is a clinical term describing a white patch.
- It has been used to describe lesions with a premalignant potential.
- Less than 10% however undergo malignant change.

WHO definition of leukoplakia

'A white patch on the oral mucosa which cannot be wiped off and is not susceptible to any other clinical diagnosis. Leukoplakia should be reserved for white patches that cannot be classified as another disease.'

Aetiological factors
The most important factors in the development of leukoplakia and oral malignancy are:
- Smoking.
- Alcohol use.
- Betel and areca nut chewing.

Symptoms
- Often symptom-free.
- If ulcerated pain is inevitably present.

Signs
- Leukoplakia has a variable appearance.
- It may be smooth, wrinkled or fissured.
- White patches may be localized affecting any part of the oral mucosa or be extensive.

- Size is not an indication of malignant potential.
- Lesions on the floor of the mouth are more commonly associated with malignant change.
- Therefore biopsy is essential to confirm the diagnosis.
- Histopathologists will check for signs of epithelial dysplasia.
- Regular monitoring and repeat biopsies may be required.
- Areas that have a speckled or erythematous appearance are considered more sinister than smooth, white patches.
- Areas of ulceration in white patches are also very significant and potentially serious signs.

13. Speckled leukoplakia

Signs
- Red lesions of the oral mucosa with small, white areas superimposed.
- Both speckled leuoplakias and erythroplakias are more likely to undergo malignant change.

14. Erythroplakia
- A bright red patch with occasional white areas.
- Usually on the buccal mucosa.
- High incidence of dysplastic change.

15. Squamous cell carcinoma (see also page 198)
- The association between oral cancer, leukoplakia and particularly speckled erythroplasia/erthroplakia is well established.
- However lesions may be present for months or years before any malignant change occurs.
- The ventral surface of the tongue and the floor of the mouth are high risk sites for malignant change.

Conclusion

- The association of white patches on oral mucosa with malignant change makes it mandatory that all such lesions are treated seriously.
- Whenever there is any uncertainty as to the diagnosis of a white patch, a biopsy is essential and practitioners may prefer to refer patients to a specialist unit for advice and treatment.

Further reading

Scully, C., Flint, S.R. and Porter, S.R. (1996) *Oral Diseases: An illustrated guide to diagnosis and management of diseases of the oral mucosa, gingivae, teeth, salivary glands, bones and joints*, 2nd edn. London: Martin Dunitz.

Soames, J.V. and Southam, J.C. (1998) *Oral Pathology*, 3rd edn. Oxford: Oxford University Press.

Lamey, P.J. and Lewis, M.A.O. (1977) *A Clinical Guide to Oral Medicine*, 2nd edn. London: British Dental Association.

12

Bumps, lumps and swellings

Summary

Introduction

History

Examination

Differential diagnosis

Developmental
Mandibular and palatal tori.
Haemangiomas and Sturge–Weber syndrome.
Lymphangiomas.
Dermoid and epidermoid cysts (see Chapter 9).
Lymphoepithelial (branchial cleft) cysts (see Chapter 9).
Thyroglossal duct cysts (see Chapter 9).
Anterior median lingual cysts (see Chapter 9).
Oral cysts with gastric or intestinal epithelium.(see Chapter 9).
Cystic hygroma (see Chapter 9).
Nasopharyngeal and thymic cysts (see Chapter 9).

Acquired

1. Traumatic
Haematoma (ecchymosis), oedema, foreign body.
Mucocele (see Chapter 9).

2. Hyperplasic
Peripheral giant cell granuloma (giant cell epulis).
Fibrous epulis.
Pregnancy epulis.
Pyogenic granuloma.
Fibro-epithelial polyp.
Denture hyperplasia.
Congenital epulis.
Drug-related hyperplasia, e.g. epanutin, cyclosporin and nifedipine (see Chapter 4).

continued

3. Infective

Bacterial
Peritonsillar abscess (quinsy).
Boil/carbuncle.
Salivary gland infection. Acute and chronic bacterial sialadenitis, salivary duct calculi.
Acute apical periodontitis of pulpal origin and apical abscess (see Chapter 5).
Acute pericoronitis (see Chapter 5).
Acute osteomyelitis (see Chapter 8).
Ludwig's angina (see Chapter 8).
Actinomycosis (see Chapter 8).
Sinus associated with chronic apical periodontitis (see Chapter 5).
Lateral periodontal abscess (see Chapter 5).
Perio-endo lesions (see Chapter 5).
Cysts, especially infected cysts (see Chapter 9).
Lymphadenopathy secondary to infection/inflammation (see Chapters 8 and 10).

Viral
Mumps, cytomegalovirus, glandular fever (see Chapter 8).
HIV associated salivary gland disease.

Fungal
Fungal infections usually present as white patches, red patches or ulcers (see Chapter 8). However, in histoplasmosis infection, mucosal nodular and vegetative lesions are described (see Chapter 10). The ulcers in patients with blastomycosis can have a warty surface, and skin pustules discharging onto the face may also be seen (see Chapter 10).

4. Neoplastic

Benign:
Epithelial: squamous cell papilloma.
Connective tissue: fibroma, lipoma, osteoma, neurofibroma, granular cell myoblastoma (granular cell tumour).
Malignant:
Epithelial: squamous cell carcinoma, verrucous carcinoma, basal cell carcinoma (rodent ulcer).
Malignant melanoma (see Chapter 10).
Connective tissue: osteosarcoma, chondrosarcoma, rhabdomyosarcoma, fibrosarcoma.
Secondary tumours.
Lymphomas, leukaemias, Kaposi's sarcoma (see Chapter 10).

continued

Salivary gland tumours
Epithelial tumours:
Benign: Pleomorphic adenoma, Warthin's tumour (adenolymphoma), basal cell adenoma, canalicular adenoma.
Malignant: Mucoepidermoid carcinoma, acinic cell carcinoma, adenoid cystic carcinoma, polymorphous low-grade adenocarcinoma.
Non-epithelial salivary gland tumours: haemangioma.
Unclassified: lymphoma, Hodgkin's disease and secondary metastatic tumours.

Odontogenic tumours
Ameloblastoma.
Adenomatoid odontogenic tumour.
Calcifying epithelial odontogenic tumour (CEOT).
Ameloblastic fibroma.
Mesenchymal tumours:
Odontogenic myxoma.
Odontogenic fibroma.

5. Miscellaneous
Fibrous dysplasia (see Chapter 13).
Paget's disease (see Chapter 13).
Sjögren's syndrome (see Chapter 13).
Angio-oedema (see Chapter 13).
Amyloid (see Chapter 13).
Systemic lupus erythematosus (see Chapter 13).
Crohn's disease (see Chapter 13).
Thyroid swellings.
Cherubism.

Introduction

Bumps, lumps and swellings in the head and neck region or mouth may be a sign of serious infection or malignancy. Alternatively they may be developmental abnormalities, e.g. mandibular or palatal tori, and require no treatment apart from reassurance of the patient. In view of the possible serious nature of any bump, lump or swelling, it is essential to establish an accurate diagnosis in order that appropriate treatment can be carried out. In all cases where malignancy is suspected, patients should be referred for specialist diagnosis and management. Patients with severe spreading infections, e.g. Ludwig's angina, will also need to be referred for admission to hospital, treatment with systemic antibiotics and appropriate surgical treatment, e.g. incision, drainage and extraction.

History

A careful, detailed history is required (see also Chapter 2) and is an essential component of the diagnosis. The following questions should be asked:

- How long have you had the bump, lump, swelling? (Present at birth or early in life, likely to be developmental. Recent onset suggests an acquired lesion.)

Important note: However, rare malignant tumours, e.g. rhabdomyosarcoma (see page 249) occur in childhood but will usually grow rapidly.

- Is it getting larger or smaller?
- Is it painful? (Pain indicates infection (e.g. abscess/cellulitis), trauma or secondary infection (of malignant tumours and cysts). Others are usually painless).
- Has there been any discharge? (Infections may discharge spontaneously, intra-orally or onto the face).
- Do you have any numbness of your lower lip or face? (Indicates a fast-growing lesion or direct nerve involvement).

Examination

Note: The examination must be thorough and methodical (see Chapter 3).

- Carefully palpate the swelling to ascertain its tissue of origin, e.g. bone, skin, lymph glands, etc.
- Record details of the size, shape and colour.
- Look at the patient's general condition. Swellings associated with recent weight loss and cachexia suggest malignancy.
- Note any tenderness, redness or warmth (indicates inflammation or infection, see Fig. 4.1, page 41).
- Assess the consistency:
  soft: e.g. lipoma, oedema.
  firm: e.g. fibrous epulis, fibro-epthelial polyp, cellulitis.
  hard: e.g. osteoma, odontogenic tumours.

rock hard: e.g. metastatic cancer.
rubbery hard: e.g. lymph glands in Hodgkin's disease.

- Check for fluctuance (see page 146). Indicates there is fluid present, e.g. abscesses and cysts in the soft tissues.
- Determine whether the swelling is fixed to the overlying skin by trying to move the skin over it. Fixation is seen in both abscesses and malignancies.

N.B. It is essential to examine relevant lymph nodes and if palpable, record details of the site, size and consistency (see page 16).

Developmental

Mandibular and palatal tori (torus mandibularis, torus palatinus)

- Hard, bony swellings of unknown aetiology.
- Rarely seen in children and grow slowly.
- Similar exostoses (bony outgrowths) are also seen in other parts of the mouth, particularly the buccal aspect of the maxilla, in the molar regions.

Symptoms

Asymptomatic unless the overlying mucosa is traumatized, when an ulcer may appear.

Signs

- A non-mobile, bony, hard swelling either in the midline of the palate or on the lingual surface of the mandible, usually in the premolar region.
- Mandibular tori are usually bilateral.

Note: Bilateral lesions are usually developmental.

- Size – extremely variable from small, flat, raised areas to large, nodular growths.

N.B. Do not normally require treatment unless they interfere with the construction of dentures.

Haemangioma

- Developmental abnormalities of blood vessels. Present at birth or early childhood.

Symptoms

- Symptom free unless traumatized, when bleeding may be extensive.

Signs
- Flat or nodular, dark red/purple swellings *which blanch on pressure*.
- Seen on the lips, tongue, buccal mucosa, cheeks and palate.
- May be divided into papillary, cavernous or mixed types depending on the size of the vascular spaces.
- May also involve muscle and bone.

N.B. It is essential to ensure that the bones of *the jaws are not involved* (using appropriate radiography and angiography, see page 68) before carrying out any dental extractions, due to the risk of serious haemorrhage. Refer if in doubt.

Sturge–Weber syndrome
A congenital disorder, presenting as haemangiomas of the face, together with oral lesions, related to the distribution of the branches of the trigeminal nerve. The meninges are also involved and patients may develop epilepsy and mental defects.

Lymphangioma
- Developmental swellings of lymph vessels.
- Less common than haemangiomas.
- Present at birth and in early childhood.
- Tongue and lips are most frequently affected.

Symptoms
- Large tongue (macroglossia).
- Large lip (macrocheilia).
- May suddenly increase in size as a result of trauma and bleeding into the lymph spaces.

Signs
- Swollen lip or tongue.
- The swelling may be soft, smooth or nodular.

Acquired

1. Traumatic (see Chapter 7)
- The cause of the trauma should be established whenever possible.
- Medico-legal reports may be required for road traffic accidents, alleged assaults, suspected child abuse, etc.
- Record all details in the patient's notes and draw diagrams or photograph to illustrate the injuries sustained.

- Traumatic bumps, lumps and swellings are usually due to either oedema or haematoma/ecchymosis (bruising).
- Oedema presents as soft, distended tissue without discoloration.
- Haematoma/ecchymosis is initially purple, from bleeding into the tissues. The swelling is firm, due to engorgement with blood, and tender. As the red blood cells are broken down, the swelling changes colour to yellow/brown.

Note: Haematomas can occur following the administration of local anaesthesia, due to trauma to blood vessels. The onset may be rapid and the size of the swelling extensive, particularly if the pterygoid plexus is traumatized. In a healthy patient with no history of bleeding disorders, it is self-limiting. The patient will need plenty of reassurance and a course of antibiotics to prevent secondary infection.

- Foreign bodies, e.g. fractured teeth, implanted in tissues, during trauma, can also cause persistent swellings. These are firm to palpation, may be tender and can be confirmed with soft tissue radiographs.

2. *Hyperplastic*

Note:

- Hyperplasia is an increase in the size of an organ or tissue due to an increase in the *number* of its cells.
- Whereas hypertrophy is an increase in the size of an organ or tissue due to an increase in the *size* of its cells, e.g. muscles in response to increased work.
- Chronic, low-grade, recurrent trauma may result in hyperplasia of oral mucosal connective tissue.
- When the gums are affected, these gingival swellings are termed epulides (singular epulis, literally 'on the gum').

Plaque and calculus are major aetiological factors in the following conditions:

i. Peripheral, giant cell granuloma **(giant cell epulis)**

- Occurs on both the gingiva and alveolar mucosa.
- Most are seen anterior to molar teeth.
- Female/male ratio is 2:1.
- Peak incidence in males is the second decade. In females it is the fifth decade.

Symptoms

- Swelling on gum which may be painful if ulcerated.

Signs
- A red, soft swelling.
- When teeth are present, usually appears interdentall buccal and lingual aspects, joined by a narrow isthmu

Diagnostic tests
- Biopsy (see page 146) and histopathological examination show a vascular lesion with multi-nucleated giant cells.
- Radiographs show superficial erosion of the interdental bone, unlike the *central giant cell granuloma* which causes more extensive bone loss and a well-defined radiolucent area.

N.B. The giant cell lesion of hyperparathyroidism (brown tumour) (see page 272) is histologically identical to the central giant cell granuloma and may also present as a soft tissue swelling.

Haematological investigations
Serum calcium, phosphorus and alkaline phosphatase levels are abnormal in hyperparathyroidism and should be requested in order to differentiate between a central giant cell granuloma and a brown tumour (see page 272).

ii. Fibrous epulis

Symptoms
- A swelling on the gum, usually pain free.

Signs
- A firm, pedunculated or sessile mass.

Note: Pedunculated – has a stalk; sessile – broad based.

- It is the same colour as the adjacent gingiva.
- Ulceration of the surface may occur due to local trauma.

Diagnosis
- Confirmed by excision biopsy and histopathological examination.

iii. Pregnancy epulis
- Onset is usually at the end of the first trimester (3 months).

Symptoms
- Soft swelling on the gum which bleeds easily (sometimes spontaneously) and may be painful due to surface ulceration.

Signs
- A red/purple coloured swelling on the gum more frequently seen in the anterior region.
- Identical histologically to the pyogenic granuloma which may occur on other sites, e.g. tongue and labial mucosa as well as the gingiva.
- Usually regress after the birth of the child.

iv. *Pyogenic granuloma*
- A vascular swelling, identical to the pregnancy epulis, histologically.
- The pyogenic granuloma was originally thought to be due to a reaction to infection by pyogenic organisms as in a similar skin lesion. Although this is *not* the case, the misnomer remains.

v. *Fibro-epithelial polyp* ~> *leaf fibroma*
- Also caused by low-grade recurrent trauma.
- Seen mainly on lips, tongue and cheeks.

Symptoms *peripheral cell granuloma, fibrous epul*
- Painless swelling. *pyogenic granuloma + pregnancy*

Signs *epulis, fibro epithelial polyp*
- Firm, pink, pedunculated or sessile swelling.
- Size varies from a few millimetres to greater than 1 centimetre in diameter.
- Becomes flattened when covered by a denture and is then termed a 'leaf fibroma'.

Diagnostic tests
- Excision biopsy and histopathological examination.

vi. *Denture hyperplasia* (Fig. 12.1)
- Associated with ill-fitting dentures.

Symptoms
- Loose, excess tissue beneath the denture.
- Painful when traumatized and ulcerated.

Signs
- Single or several folds of pink tissue in the sulcus related to the periphery of a denture.
- Dentures are usually ill-fitting and worn.

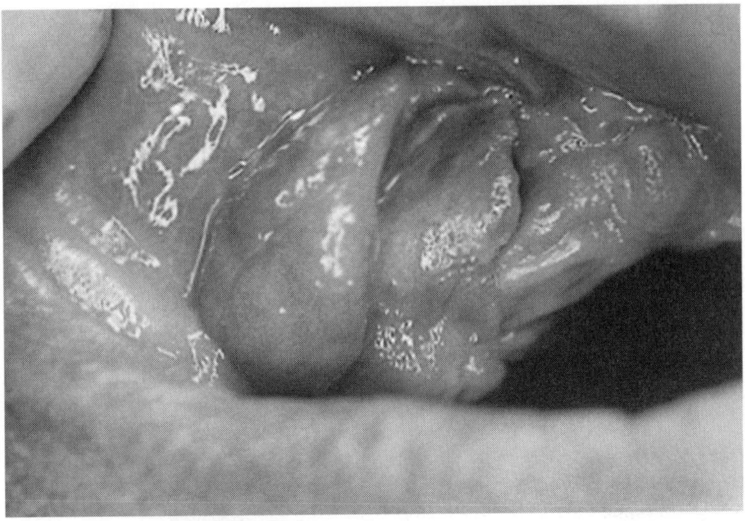

Figure 12.1 Denture hyperplasia.

- The lower jaw is more frequently affected than the upper due to the reduced area for support and increased instability of lower dentures.

Diagnostic tests
- Excision biopsy and histopathological examination.
- Histologically similar to the fibro-epithelial polyp.
- Patients presenting with multiple folds of denture hyperplasia (Fig. 12.1), a should be referred to a maxillofacial/oral surgery consultant for excision of the hyperplastic tissue and soft tissue grafting if required, prior to the construction of new dentures.

***vii. Congenital epulis* (gingival granular cell tumour)**
- Rare. Seen in newborn infants as a pedunculated, nodular swelling.
- Usually occurs in the maxillary, anterior region.
- Female to male ratio, 10:1.

Diagnostic tests
- Excision biopsy and histopathological examination.

3. *Infective*

i. Peritonsillar abscess (quinsy)

Aetiology

- Infection from a tonsillar crypt or the supratonsillar fossa.
- May also be caused by spread of infection (pericoronitis) from a lower third molar (see pages 94–96).

Symptoms

- Pain.
- Difficulty swallowing (dysphagia).
- Sore throat.
- Fever.

Signs

- Cervical lymphadenopathy.
- Pyrexia (raised temperature).
- Possible trismus (limitation of opening).
- Uvula is displaced.
- Tongue is coated and there is marked halitosis.
- Swollen and erythematous, tonsillar, faucial and soft palate regions.

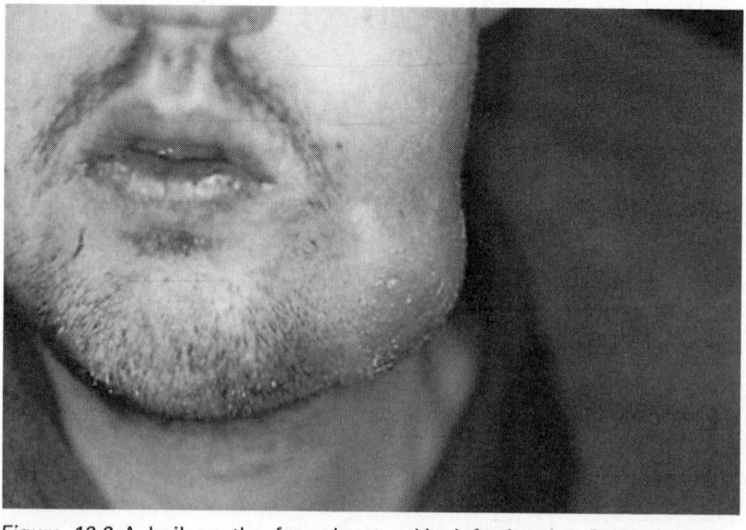

Figure 12.2 A boil on the face due to skin infection by *Staphylococcus aureus.*

- Swelling may extend across the midline.
- Substantial narrowing of oropharynx.

N.B. Patients with peritonsillar abscesses should be immediately referred to either a maxillofacial surgeon or an ear, nose and throat department for treatment, which involves drainage and antibiotics, as further spread of infection may lead to the airway being compromised.

***ii. Boil/carbuncle* (Fig. 12.2)**

A skin infection caused by *Staphylococcus aureus*.

Symptoms

- A painful swelling on the face or neck.

Signs

- A tender, warm, erythematous swelling of the skin which can be moved on the underlying tissues, e.g. the mandible.
- Fluctuance can be demonstrated (see page 146) if pus has collected.

N.B. Can be differentiated from a dental infection as:

- There is no history of dental pain/toothache.
- There is no intra-oral associated dental pathology.
- There is no tenderness of any teeth to percussion or dull percussion note (see page 38) and there are no radiographic signs of a dental aetiology.
- It is therefore important that the patient is referred to their general medical practitioner for appropriate antibiotic therapy and also for drainage of the swelling should pus collect.

Salivary gland infection

- Salivary gland swelling may occur as a result of viral infections, e.g. mumps, cytomegalovirus (see page 51) and HIV.
- They may also be enlarged in Sjögren's syndrome (see page 277), sarcoidosis and when there is neoplastic change, either benign or malignant (see next section of this chapter).

Examination of the major salivary glands is described on page 17.

Bacterial infection is usually caused by either oral streptococci, *Staphylococcus aureus* or oral anaerobes. Two forms of bacterial infection have been described.

i. Acute bacterial sialadenitis

- Predisposing factors are salivary duct calculi, dehydration and debilitated patients, e.g. following major abdominal surgery.

- Aetiology is thought to be due to reduced salivary flow.
- Also occurs in patients with Sjögren's syndrome and with xerostomia (dry mouth) from other causes, e.g. drug or radiation therapy.

Symptoms
- Painful, swollen, salivary gland.

Signs
- Dry mouth.
- Tenderness and possibly redness of the skin overlying the affected gland.
- Malaise.
- Pyrexia.
- Pus may be seen intra-orally or expressed from the affected duct when the gland is massaged.

Diagnosis
- Culture and antibiotic sensitivity of any pus expressed.
- Following resolution of acute symptoms with antibiotic therapy, sialography is indicated to assess the patency of the duct system and the integrity of the acinar structure of the gland.

ii. Chronic bacterial sialadenitis
- A low-grade inflammatory condition usually associated with obstruction of the salivary duct.
- The submandibular gland is more frequently affected than the parotid.
- Exacerbation leads to acute bacterial sialadenitis.
- Usually unilateral.

Symptoms
- Recurrent, tender swelling of the affected gland.
- An unpleasant salty taste in the mouth.

Signs
- An enlarged, tender salivary gland.
- During acute exacerbations, pus may be expressed from the duct if the gland is massaged.

Diagnostic tests
- Sialography

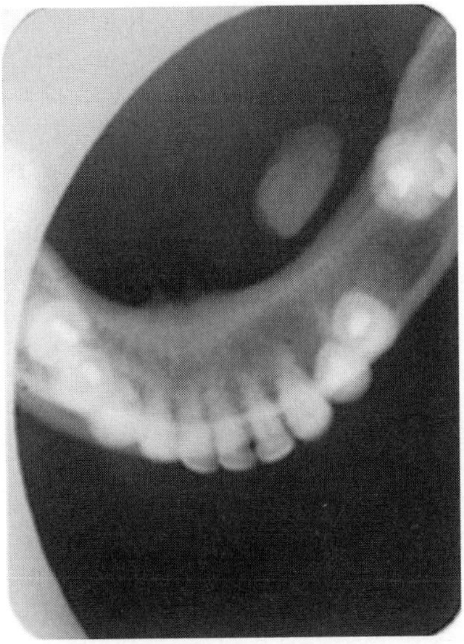

Figure 12.3 Salivary duct calculus.

iii. Salivary duct calculi

The most common cause of acute and recurrent swelling of the salivary glands in adults is the presence of salivary calculi (sialoliths) obstructing the outflow of saliva by blocking the duct of the gland.

- The submandibular gland is more frequently involved.
- Usually unilateral.
- Multiple stones may occur in the same gland or duct.
- Blockage of salivary flow leads to acute infection and may cause chronic inflammatory changes in the gland itself.

Symptoms
- Pain.
- Swelling of the gland, particularly at meals times when salivary flow is stimulated.

Signs
- Tender, enlarged salivary gland.
- The calculus may be visible in the duct and appears as a yellow or white coloured stone.
- Calculi may also be palpable in the submandibular duct (see page 17) and at the orifice of the parotid duct.

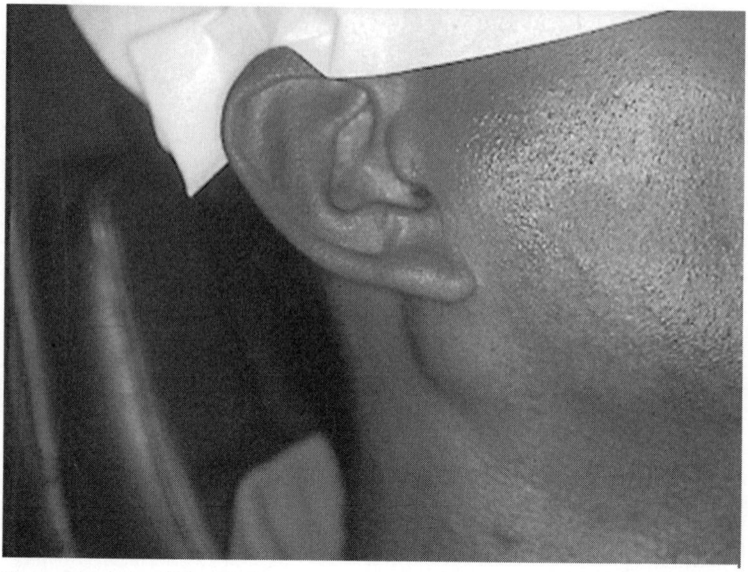

Figure 12.4 Swelling of the parotid gland due to HIV associated salivary gland disease.

Diagnostic tests (Fig. 12.3)

- Radiographs confirm the presence of radiopaque stones.
- A lower occlusal should be used for the submandibular duct and a film placed in the cheek for the parotid gland.
- Sialography will confirm the stricture and obstruction caused by the calculus.
- Ultrasound will demonstrate the presence of an obstruction.

iv. HIV associated salivary gland disease

- A group II lesion (less commonly associated with HIV infection) (see page 153).
- Seen in both children and adults (rarely), infected with HIV.
- Presents as swelling of the parotid gland (Fig. 12.4).

Symptoms

- Painless, unilateral or bilateral parotid swellings.
- Xerostomia (dry mouth) may be present.
- Dry mouth may also occur without swelling of the salivary glands in HIV infected patients.

Signs
- A firm, painless swelling of the parotid gland.
- Young adults and children affected (in contrast with Sjögren's syndrome) (see page 277).
- Generalized lymphadenopathy may be present.

Diagnostic tests
- CT scanning shows multiple cystic change within the parotid glands, usually bilaterally.
- Labial gland biopsy may show lymphocytic infiltration.
- Other oral changes (see page 277) associated with HIV infection may also be seen.
- HIV antibody testing after appropriate counselling may be indicated.

4. *Neoplastic*

Benign

Epithelial tumours

i. Squamous cell papilloma
- Usually a solitary lesion seen on the palate, but can occur anywhere on the oral mucosa.
- Associated with the human papilloma virus (HPV).

Symptoms
- A painless swelling.

Signs
- May be pedunculated or sessile.
- Classically described as a cauliflower-like growth with a white or pink surface depending on the degree of keratinization.
- Dysplasia is not seen histologically and the squamous cell papilloma does not undergo malignant change.

Diagnostic tests
- Excision biopsy and histopathology.

Connective tissue benign tumours

i. Fibroma
- As with other connective tumours of the oral cavity, less common than the hyperplastic lesions.
- Clinically identical in appearance to the fibro-epithelial polyp.

Symptoms

- A painless swelling.

Signs

- A firm, pink, pedunculated or sessile swelling, most frequently seen on the palate or gingiva.

Diagnostic tests

- Excision biopsy and histopathological examination.

ii. Lipoma

- A benign tumour of mature adipose (fat) cells.
- Rare intra-orally.

Symptoms

- A painless, soft swelling most frequently seen on the cheek, buccal mucosa, lips and floor of the mouth.

Signs

- A yellow, soft, mobile swelling which may *appear* fluctuant (pseudo-fluctuation).

Diagnostic tests

- Excision biopsy and histopathological examination.

iii. Osteoma

- A benign, slow-growing tumour of bone.

Symptoms

- A painless, hard swelling which slowly increases in size.

Signs

- A bony, hard swelling usually solitary.
- Multiple osteomas occur in Gardner's syndrome. This is a rare familial disorder transmitted as an autosomal dominant trait. It comprises: *multiple jaw osteomas*, epidermoid cysts, lipomas, fibromas, pigmented ocular fundic lesions and multiple polyps in the colon, which have a high potential for malignant change. There may also be impacted supernumerary teeth. *All patients with multiple osteomas* must be referred for a complete intestinal evaluation in view of the risk of malignant disease.
- Osteomas can be divided into compact or cancellous varieties.
- Usually seen at the angle of the mandible.
- The location helps to differentiate osteomas from tori.

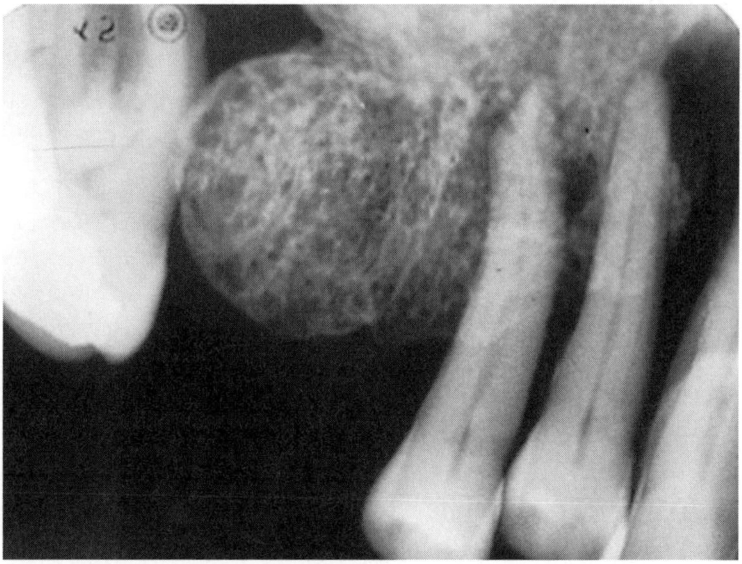

Figure 12.5 Osteoma in the right maxillary first molar region.

Diagnostic tests

- Radiology shows a well-circumscribed radiopaque lesion (Fig. 12.5).
- Biopsy and histopathology.

Tumours of peripheral nerves

iv. Neurofibroma

- Seen in von Recklinghausen's disease (multiple neurofibromatosis) as multiple tumours.
- May also be solitary.
- A developmental disorder of nerve sheaths.
- Can be inherited as an autosomal dominant trait.
- Malignant change to sarcoma is seen in multiple neurofibromatosis in approximately 5–15% of cases.
- Malignant change in solitary lesions is very rare.
- Skin swellings may cause extensive disfigurement (elephantiasis neuromatosa)
- Complications include mental handicap, epilepsy and paraplegia due to central and spinal involvement.
- Uncommon in the mouth (approximately 5% of cases).
- Skin tumours develop at puberty.

Symptoms
- Usually painless, soft tissue swellings of the tongue and gingiva.
- Skin lesions may cause itching.
- When associated with the inferior dental and other nerves in the head and neck region, facial pain, deafness and paraesthesia (altered sensation) may occur.
- Skin pigmentation (café-au-lait) spots may be present. These develop early in life and precede the skin tumours.

Signs
- Multiple, maybe hundreds, of soft swellings.
- Anywhere on the body may be affected.
- In the mouth, soft, pedunculated swellings are seen.
- These may be sessile on the gum.
- Tumours are mobile laterally but *not* mobile in the line of the nerve.

Diagnostic tests
- Isolated lesions can be excised and the specimens sent for histopathological examination.
- Multiple lesions such as seen in von Recklinghausen's disease, should be treated only when causing symptoms or when they are particularly unsightly, as excision of all growths is impractical.
- Radiographs (panoral) may show cyst-like radiolucent areas when bones are involved.

N.B. Patients must be reviewed by their medical practitioner or dermatologist, as well as their dental practitioner, when oral lesions are present, in view of the high incidence of malignant transformation.

v. Granular cell myoblastoma (granular cell tumour)
- Thought to be of neural origin.

Symptoms
- A painless swelling most commonly seen in the tongue.

Signs
- A firm, non-tender swelling with a smooth surface and grey/white colour.

Diagnostic tests
- Excision biopsy and histopathology.

vi. Ossifying fibroma (cemento-ossifying fibroma)

- A well circumscribed lesion of the jaws consisting of fibrous tissue, bone and other mineralized tissue resembling cementum. Similar histologically to fibrous dysplasia (see page 276), from which it can be differentiated, as it is well demarcated, in contrast to lesions of fibrous dysplasia which are ill-defined and merge with normal bone.
- Usually seen between 20 and 40 years of age.

Symptoms

- A painless, slow-growing swelling of the jaws.
- Most commonly seen in the premolar/molar regions of the mandible.

Signs

- A non-tender, hard swelling usually expanding both buccal and lingual cortical plates.

Diagnostic tests

Radiology

- A well-demarcated, radiolucent lesion with a circumscribed radiopaque margin.
- Within the lesion calcified radiopaque material is present.
- Although usually slow growing, in some children and adolescents there may be rapid growth.
- The recurrence rate of fast-growing lesions, in adolescents and children can be as high as 60%.
- Biopsy and histopathological examination are also required.

Malignant

Epithelial

i. Squamous cell carcinoma

See also Chapter 10, page 198. Varied clinical presentation.

Symptoms

- Can occur as a painless swelling.
- Or as an area of ulceration, which is initially painless but can cause severe pain if nerve involvment occurs or when infected.
- May also present as a red (erythroplakia) or white (leukoplakia) patch.

Signs

- A swelling which is indurated (abnormal hardening of an organ or tissue) and fixed to underlying structures.

- When the tongue is involved, its mobility is reduced as the tongue becomes fixed to the floor of the mouth.
- Essential to palpate the regional lymph nodes (see page 16), as 30% of patients have lymph node involvement at presentation.
- Enlarged nodes become firm or hard, are non tender and may also be fixed to the adjacent tissue.

ii. Verrucous carcinoma

- A slow-growing, low-grade, squamous cell carcinoma occurring on the oral mucosa and also on the skin.
- Locally invasive, it is most commonly found in the buccal sulcus of tobacco chewers.

Symptoms

- Usually painless.
- A thickened, white, warty, swelling.

Signs

- Thick, white folds of epithelial tissue.
- A warty, cauliflower-like, lesion.
- Does not metastasize.

Diagnosis

- Biopsy and histopathology.

N.B. Treatment for verrucous carcinoma is surgical as there have been reports of malignant changes in lesions treated with radiotherapy.

iii. Basal cell carcinoma/rodent ulcer

- A tumour of skin.
- Does not occur in the mouth.
- Seen in the elderly, particularly those with outdoor occupations or Europeans living in hot climates.
- Ultraviolet radiation and sunlight are major aetiological factors.
- Multiple naevoid basal cell carcinomas and odontogenic keratocysts are a feature of the multiple basal cell naevous syndrome (Gorlin and Goltz syndrome).

Symptoms

- A painless, slow-growing swelling on the face or lip.

Signs

- A raised, nodular swelling that may be ulcerated. The margins are *raised, rolled and pearly*.

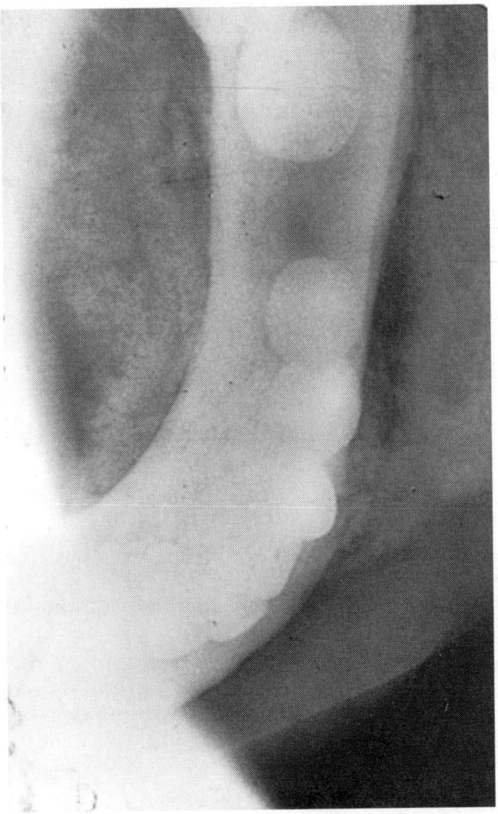

Figure 12.6
Osteosarcoma of the body of the left mandible.

- Locally invasive and destructive. Metastatic spread is very rare.

Diagnosis
- Excision biopsy and histopathology.

Connective tissue

i. Osteosarcoma (Fig. 12.6).
- The most common primary malignant tumour of bone.
- As with other sarcomas tends to metastasize via the blood rather than the lymphatics.
- However, it rarely affects the jaws.
- More common in the mandible.
- Males more frequently affected than females.
- Usually occurs between 30 and 40 years of age.

- May present as a complication of Paget's disease or radiotherapy.
- A rapidly invasive tumour with high recurrence rate.

Symptoms
- A rapidly growing, painful swelling.
- Firm or hard.
- Limited jaw opening.
- Numbness of the lower lip.
- Loose teeth.

Signs
- A firm or hard swelling of the jaw.
- Trismus.
- Ulceration of the mucosa is a late sign.
- Abnormal tooth mobility.

Diagnostic tests
Radiology (Fig. 12.6)
- Variable appearance with irregular bone destruction presenting as radiolucencies in tumours which are mainly radiopaque due to the formation of neoplastic bone.
- When the periosteum is raised, following perforation of the cortical plates, the appearance of the perpendicular bony trabeculae is given the name 'sunray'.
- Biopsy and histopathological examination.

Rare connective tissue tumours of the jaws include:

ii. Chondrosarcoma
- Most common site is the anterior part of the maxilla (approximately 60% of cases).

Symptoms
- Pain, swelling, loosening of teeth.

Signs
- A firm or hard swelling.
- Drifting and mobility of teeth.

Diagnostic tests
Radiology
- Radiographs show a multilocular and poorly circumscribed radiolucency.

Biopsy and histopathological examination

- Can be difficult to distinguish between malignant and benign tumours.
- Chondrosarcomas rarely metastasize but local recurrences are common and may be more aggressive than the original tumour.

iii. Rhabdomyosarcoma
- A malignant tumour of striated muscle.
- Rare in the oral cavity, but the most common soft tissue sarcoma of the head and neck.
- Seen in children *under* 10 years old.

Symptoms
- A painless swelling, usually of the soft palate.

Signs
- A rapidly growing soft swelling.
- May present as multiple polyp-like swellings which resemble a bunch of grapes (botryoid rhabdomyosarcoma).

Diagnostic tests
- Biopsy and histopathological examination.

iv. Fibrosarcoma
- Very rarely seen in the jaws and oral soft tissues.
- Most occur in the mandible and in adults.
- Can also occur on the tongue and cheeks.
- Most patients 30–55 years of age.

Symptoms
- Swellings may have variable growth rate.
- Pain occurs with ulceration and secondary infection/haemorrhage.

Signs
- A smooth, lobulated, firm swelling.
- May be bulky and fleshy due to the proliferation of collagen and fibroblasts.
- There may be surface ulceration.

Diagnostic tests
- Biopsy and histopathological examination.

v. Secondary tumours
- Occur in the jaws, usually the angle of the mandible, as a result of metastatic spread via the blood stream.
- Tumours which metastasize to the jaws most commonly are *lung (bronchus), breast, prostate, thyroid and kidney.*

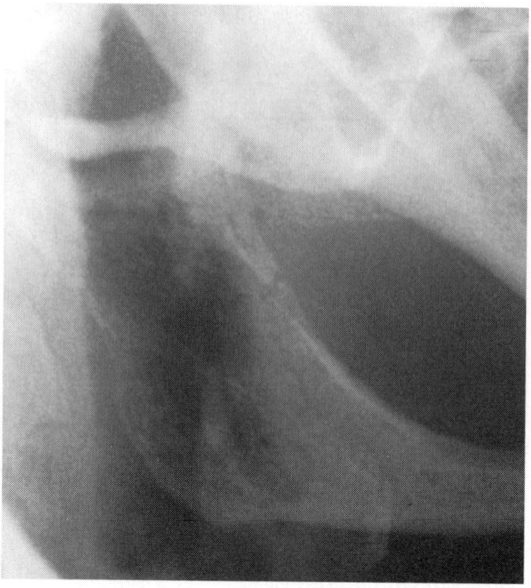

Figure 12.7 Secondary tumour in the ascending ramus of the mandible.

- They may be the first clinical presentation of an undiagnosed primary tumour.

Symptoms
- Pain, swelling and numbness of the lower lip when the inferior alveolar nerve is involved.
- Loosening of teeth.
- May also present as a soft tissue swelling in a recent extraction site, when the tumour herniates into the socket.

Signs
- Typically an elderly patient with a firm or hard facial/oral swelling.
- Intra-orally may occur as a soft irregular, red or purple swelling arising from a tooth socket.

Diagnostic tests
Radiology (Fig. 12.7)
- An irregular radiolucency which may be extensive.
- Typically a motheaten appearance which resembles osteomyelitis.

- Secondary tumours from the prostate, however, are usually sclerotic (radiopaque).

Biopsy and histopathological examination

- If secondary metastatic tumour is confirmed, the patient must be referred for a comprehensive medical, radiographical and haematological examination in order to determine the site of the primary tumour.

Salivary gland tumours

(For examination of the parotid and submandibular glands see Chapter 3, page 17).,

- Classified by the World Health Organisation into epithelial tumours, non-epithelial tumours and unclassified tumours.
- 80% of salivary gland tumours occur in the parotid gland.
- 80% are benign.
- Pain and rapid growth are the symptoms which suggest malignancy, though infections and adenolymphomas (Warthin's tumour) can also be painful.

Benign tumours of salivary glands

Epithelial tumours

i. Pleomorphic adenoma

- The commonest salivary gland tumour.
- Accounts for 65% of parotid tumours, 60% of submandibular tumours and 45% of tumours of minor salivary glands.
- Rarely seen in the sublingual gland.
- Females are more frequently affected.
- The majority occur between 50 and 60 years of age.
- Minor gland tumours occur on the palate, lips and buccal mucosa.

Symptoms

- A painless, slow-growing swelling that the patient may be aware of for several years.

Signs

- A soft or rubbery swelling that may feel lobulated.
- Intra-orally the swellings are mobile on deeper tissues.
- The overlying skin or mucosa is normal unless traumatized.

Diagnostic tests

- Fine-needle aspiration to obtain a sample of tissue (see page 49) and microscopic examination of the cells.

- Computerized tomography (CT scan) shows a lobulated appearance of the tumour and distinguishes between glandular and adjacent soft tissue.
- Magnetic resonance imaging (MRI).
- Sialography is useful for chronic inflammatory changes but is of little value in diagnosing tumours.

N.B. Although a benign tumour, infiltration of the capsule, which can show variations in thickness, is common.

- Excisional biopsy of parotid tumours is *contraindicated* due to the risk of spreading the tumour cells.

NB. The tumours are often mucinous in consistency and can burst easily.

- This results in multiple recurrences.
- Malignant change may occur, though it is uncommon and more likely in recurrences.

ii. Warthin's tumour (adenolymphoma)

- A benign tumour of the parotid gland.
- Slow growing.
- Male to female ratio 3:2.
- May be bilateral (10%) or multifocal in a single gland. Most patients are over 50 years old.

Symptoms

- A painless swelling usually, though some may cause pain due to the cystic nature of the tumour.

Signs

A soft swelling of the parotid gland.

Diagnostic tests

- As for pleomorphic adenoma.

iii. Basal cell adenoma

- 75% are found in the parotid glands and 20% in the upper lip.
- 1% of all salivary tumours.

Signs, symptoms and diagnostic tests

- As for other benign salivary tumours.

iv. Canalicular adenomas.

- Most patients over 50 years.
- Presents as a painless swelling of the *upper lip*.

Diagnostic tests
- Excision biopsy and histopathology.

Other rare benign salivary gland tumours

Include ductal papillomas, clear cell adenomas, oncocytomas and papillary cystadenomas.

Malignant tumours of salivary glands
- Carcinomas of salivary glands are relatively uncommon.
- Approximately 1% of all malignancies.

N.B. Tumours of the submandibular, sublingual and minor salivary glands are more likely to be *malignant* than those in the parotid.

- Symptoms of pain, rapid growth, swollen lymph glands and facial palsy (in parotid tumours) are indicative of malignancy.
- Fixation to adjacent tissues is a further clinical sign.

i. Mucoepidermoid carcinomas
- Most occur in the parotid gland and account for 1.5% of parotid tumours.
- Relative incidence is in fact higher in the minor salivary glands, 10–15% of tumours, with the palate being the most frequent site.
- *Never* seen in sublingual glands.
- Highest incidence between 40 and 50 years of age.

Symptoms
- May be identical clinically to a benign, pleomorphic adenoma.
- However, may cause pain, ulceration and facial nerve weakness (see page 64).

Signs
- Cystic tumours may be fluctuant.
- Mucosal ulceration may be present.
- Facial nerve palsy may be seen with parotid mucoepidermoid carcinomas.

Diagnostic tests
- CT scanning and MRI.
- Histopathological examination confirms the diagnosis and enables the tumours to be graded as well-differentiated (low-grade) and poorly differentiated (high-grade) types.
- High-grade tumours have recurrence rates of as high as 80% and a 5-year survival rate of 40%.

- Low-grade tumours have a recurrence rate of less than 10% and a 5-year survival of 95%.

ii. Acinic cell carcincoma

- 85% found in the parotid gland.
- Rarely seen in the submandibular or sublingual glands.
- Female to male ratio 2:1.
- Peak incidence in patients over 70.

Signs and symptoms

- As for benign adenomas, though poorly differentiated tumours may cause facial palsy.

Diagnostic tests

- As for pleomorphic adenomas.
- Histopathological examination confirms the diagnosis.

iii Adenoid cystic carcinoma

- Usually seen in patients of 60 years and above.
- 70% of adenoid cystic carcinomas occur in the submandibular and minor salivary glands.
- Account for 30% of minor salivary gland tumours.

Symptoms

- Pain and ulceration of skin or mucosa are more common than in pleomorphic adenomas.
- Facial palsy is frequent in parotid tumours.
- Usually slow growing, however, and may be indistinguishable clinically from the pleomorphic adenoma.

Diagnostic tests

- As described previously.
- Histological examination confirms the diagnosis as the adenoid cystic carcinoma has a characteristic 'Swiss cheese' appearance.

N.B.

- The spread of this tumour along and around nerves is a typical feature (perineural and intraneural spread).
- Dissemination also occurs along the marrow spaces and bony canals.
- Metastasizes late to regional lymph nodes and lungs.

iv. Polymorphous low-grade adenocarcinoma

- Occurs in the minor salivary glands particularly the palate.

Symptoms
- A painless palatal swelling.

Signs
- A firm swelling which may later ulcerate.
- Tumours are locally invasive.
- They rarely metastasize.
- Other varieties of salivary carcinomas have been described including adenocarcinomas (not otherwise specified), salivary duct carcinomas, squamous cell carcinomas, basal cell adenocarcinomas and undifferentiated carcinomas.
- Clinical signs and symptoms are the same as the other malignant salivary tumours.
- Diagnosis is confirmed by histopathological examination.

Non-epithelial tumours
- *Less than 5%* of salivary gland tumours are non-epithelial.

Haemangioma
- May be present at birth.
- Seen in young children.

Symptoms
- A painless swelling of the parotid gland.

Signs
- A soft, sometimes blue, swelling of the parotid.

Unclassified tumours

i. Lymphoma
- Primary lymphomas of salivary glands are rare.
- Usually a part of disseminated disease.
- Parotid glands most commonly affected.
- Also seen in submandibular and minor salivary glands in the palate.
- Patients 50 years of age or more.
- Female to male ratio 2:1.
- A complication of Sjögren's syndrome (5% of patients) and benign lympho-epithelial lesion (BLL) which has the same histological appearance as Sjögren's syndrome.

Symptoms
- A painful, fast-growing swelling.
- Facial nerve weakness when the parotid gland is involved.

Signs
- A firm swelling of the gland.
- Fixation to adjacent structures is a late sign.
- Facial nerve weakness may be present.

Diagnostic tests
- As described previously.
- Histopathology confirms that most are non-Hodgkin's type.

ii. Hodgkin's disease
- Rarely affects salivary glands.
- Male to female ratio 4:1.
- Peak incidence 30–40 years of age.

Symptoms
- A painless swelling of the salivary gland.

Signs
- A soft, *rubbery* swelling which may be due to disease in the adjacent cervical lymph nodes rather than the glands themselves.

Diagnostic tests
- As above

iii. Secondary metastatic tumours
- Rare in the salivary glands.
- Most are in fact secondary deposits in adjacent lymph nodes.
- Most common primary tumours are melanomas and skin tumours.

Odontogenic tumours

i. Ameloblastoma
- A tumour of odontogenic epithelium.
- Comparatively rare and slow growing.
- Less than 1% of all oral tumours.
- Most diagnosed in patients between 30 and 60 years of age but can occur in children and the elderly.
- 80% develop in the mandible, 70% of these in the molar region and ascending ramus.
- May be first discovered as an incidental finding on radiograph.

Symptoms
- Symptom free in the early stages.
- As the tumour increases in size, a hard swelling, due to expansion of the jaw, occurs.

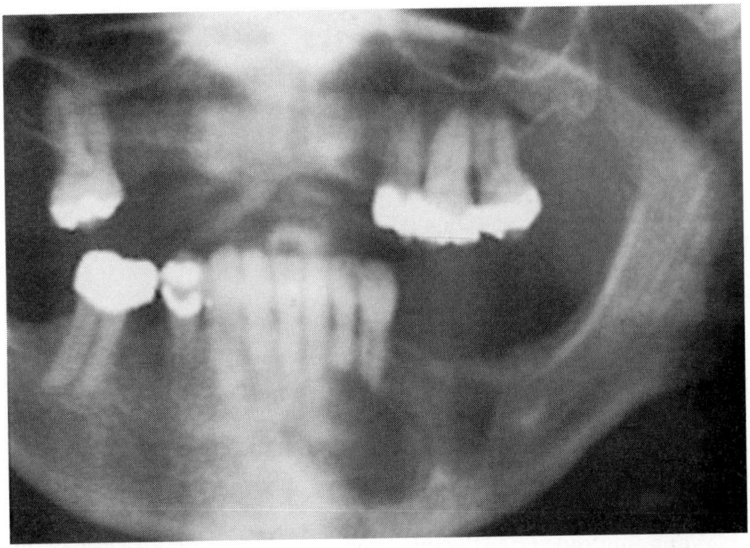

Figure 12.8 Ameloblastoma in left mandibular canine premolar region.

- Facial deformity with large tumours.
- Rarely may cause pain or paraesthesia.
- Loose teeth.

Signs
- A bony, hard, non-tender swelling of the jaw.
- 'Egg-shell crackling' (see page 163) may be associated with large tumours due to thinning of the bone.
- Eventually the bone may be perforated with extension into the adjacent soft tissues.
- Teeth may be mobile.

Diagnostic tests
- Radiology (Fig 12.8).
- A *multiloculated* radiolucency usually, but 10% may be unicystic.
- If associated with unerupted teeth may resemble a dentigerous cyst.
- Bony margins are scalloped.
- Roots of adjacent teeth are often resorbed ('mice nibbles').
- An occlusal view is of benefit, in addition to the panoral, as this may show buccal and lingual plate expansion.

- Other variants include a 'soap-bubble' or 'honeycomb' appearance of the bone on radiograph.

Biopsy and histopathological examination
- Two types are described, the follicular and flexiform, both of which contain stellate reticulum-like cells.
- Cyst formation is common.
- Ameloblastomas are locally invasive and require wide excision to avoid recurrence.

N.B.
- Unicystic ameloblastomas occur in younger patients (20–30 years) and in the mandibular third molar regions.
- Identical to dentigerous cysts on radiograph and usually associated with unerupted third molars.
- Diagnosis is confirmed by histopathological examination.
- May be treated successfully by enucleation and curettage rather than wide excision.

ii. Adenomatoid odontogenic tumour (formerly known as an adenoameloblastoma)
- More common in females. Ratio 2:1.
- A benign tumour usually seen in patients 20–30 years of age.
- Found in the *canine region of the maxilla.*

Symptoms
- A slow-growing, painless, swelling.

Signs
- A hard swelling of the maxilla.

Diagnostic tests
Radiology
- Shows a well-defined radiolucency.
- Calcification within the tumour may appear as radiopacities.

N.B. Important to differentiate from the ameloblastoma as the adenomatoid odontogenic tumour needs enucleation only and does not recur.

iii. Calcifying epithelial odontogenic tumour (CEOT)
- Also known as the Pindborg tumour.
- A rare, benign but locally invasive tumour.
- Average age of patients 40 years.
- *Mandible* affected twice as frequently as the maxilla.
- Most occur in the molar or premolar region.

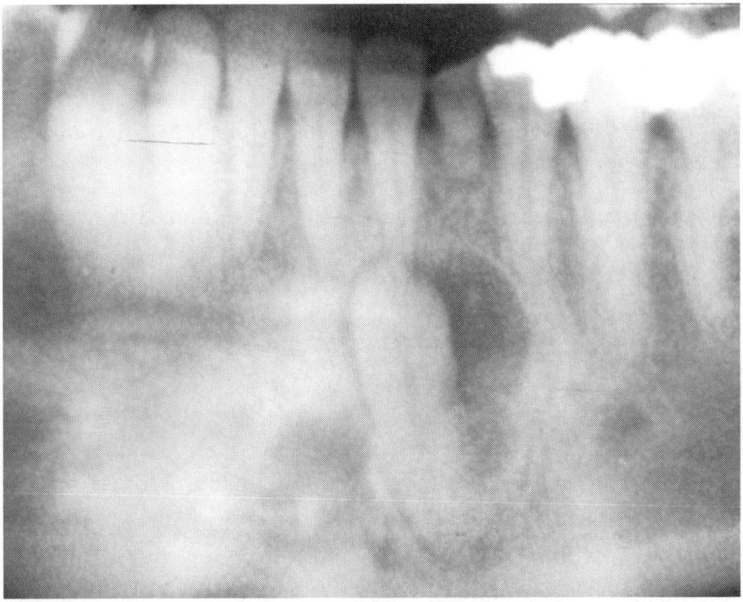

Figure 12.9 Calcifying epithelial odontogenic tumour in mandibular incisor and canine region.

- Often associated with an unerupted tooth.

Symptoms
- A painless, bony, hard swelling.

Diagnostic tests
Radiology (Fig. 12.9)
- An irregular radiolucency with ill-defined margins.
- Within the radiolucency there are radiopaque areas due to calcification.
- May be associated with the crown of an unerupted tooth.

Biopsy and histopathological examination
- Confirms amyloid-like deposits and multinucleated giant cells.
- May resemble a poorly differentiated carcinoma, from which it must be distinguished.

iv. Ameloblastic fibroma
- A rare, benign tumour affecting young adults.
- Important to differentiate from the ameloblastoma as it is not locally invasive.

Symptoms
- A slow-growing, painless swelling.

Signs
- A hard swelling usually in the *premolar or molar region of the mandible.*

Diagnostic tests
Radiology
- A unilocular or multilocular radiolucency.

Biopsy and histopathological examination
- Some lesions may contain dentine and are called 'ameloblastic fibro-dentinomas'.

Other rare odontogenic tumours described in the literature include:

Squamous odontogenic tumours, odontoameloblastomas, malignant ameloblastomas, ameloblastic carcinomas and clear cell odontogenic carcinomas.

Tumours of mesenchymal origin

i. Odontogenic myxoma
- A benign tumour of odontogenic mesenchyme.
- Affects *young adults* and growth may be rapid at first.
- Locally invasive and requires wide excision.
- Due to local infiltration, recurrence is common.
- There is frequently a tooth missing in the area of the tumour.

Symptoms
- A painless swelling of the jaw.
- Loose teeth.

Signs
- A firm or hard swelling.
- Tooth mobility when roots of the teeth are affected.

Diagnostic tests
Radiology
- A multiloculated radiolucency with a 'soap bubble' appearance. Similar radiographically to the ameloblastoma.
- Roots of adjacent teeth may show resorption.

Biopsy and histopathology
- Required to confirm the diagnosis.

ii. Odontogenic fibroma

- A rare, benign tumour.
- More common in the mandible.
- Does not infiltrate and can be treated by simple excision.

Symptoms

- A painless, slow-growing jaw swelling.

Signs

- A firm or hard swelling.

Diagnostic tests

Radiology

- A well-defined unilocular radiolucency in the tooth-bearing areas of the jaw.
- Biopsy and histopathological examination confirms the diagnosis.

5. *Miscellaneous*

Cherubism

- An autosomal dominant, inherited disease.
- Twice as common in males.
- Symmetrical swellings of the mandible characteristically appear between 2 and 4 years of age.
- Usually the angle of the mandible is involved.
- Swellings enlarge during childhood and then regress.
- Maxillary involvement causes fullness of the cheeks and a plump face, giving the characteristic cherub appearance.

Symptoms

- Painless swellings of the jaws.
- Extensive mandibular swelling may cause problems with speech and swallowing.
- Teeth may be displaced and loose.

Signs

- *Symmetrical*, firm or hard mandibular and facial swellings.
- Plumpness of the face.
- Sclera below the iris become visible due to maxillary lesions displacing the orbital floor.
- Submandibular lymphadenopathy due to reactive hyperplasia.
- Premature loss of deciduous teeth.
- Unerupted permanent teeth.
- Failure of the development of permanent teeth.
- Displaced teeth.

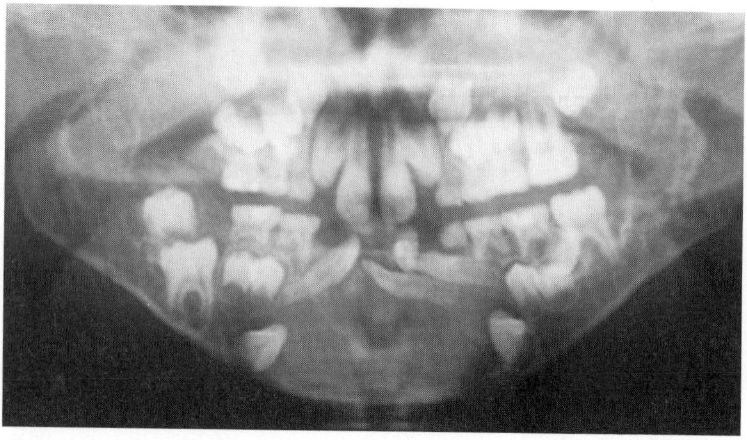

Figure 12.10 Cherubism; multilocular bilateral radiolucencies at the angle of the mandible, displaced and missing teeth.

Diagnostic tests

Radiology (Fig. 12.10)

- Multilocular radiolucencies.
- Bilateral lesions involving the angles of the mandible.
- May resemble multilocular cysts.
- Involvement of the sinuses may appear as radiopacities.

Biopsy and histopathology

- Show multinucleated giant cells in a vascular fibrous tissue stroma. May be distinguished from fibrous dysplasia by:
- The presence of giant cells on biopsy.
- The symmetrical appearance of the lesions.
- Earlier onset.
- A family history of cherubism.
- As the condition is self-limiting, treatment is required only for extensive lesions which may require conservative cosmetic surgery. This should be delayed until adolescence, when the condition becomes quiescent.

Further reading

Cawson, R.A., Langdon, J.D. and Eveson, J.W. (1996) *Surgical Pathology of the Mouth and Jaws*, 1st edn. Oxford: Wright.

Soames, J.V. and Southam, J.C. (1998) *Oral Pathology*, 3rd edn. Oxford: Oxford University Press.

Seward, G.R., Harris, M., McGowan, D.A., Killey, H.C. and Kay, L.W. (1998) *An Outline of Oral Surgery: Parts I and II*. Oxford: Wright.

13

Oral changes in systemic disease

Summary

Introduction

Differential diagnosis

1. **Vitamins**
   A
   B complex
   C
   D
   E
   K
2. **Endocrine**
   Pregnancy
   Pituitary
   Thyroid
   Parathyroid
   Pancreas (diabetes mellitus)
   Adrenal glands
3. **Gastrointestinal**
   Ulcerative colitis
   Crohn's disease
4. **Bone**
   Paget's disease
   Fibrous dysplasia
5. **Immunologically mediated**
   Sjögren's syndrome
   Angio-oedema
   Amyloid
   Systemic lupus erythematosus
6. **Haematological**
   Anaemia
   Jaundice
   Leukaemia
   Thrombocytopenia

Introduction

Although most changes in the oral cavity are due to local disease processes, many systemic conditions can present as changes within the mouth or may influence the progression of dental disease and patient management. Systemic diseases will be considered under the following headings:

1. Vitamins

Vitamin A deficiency

- Found in animal fats, milk and liver.
- Also present as carotenes in vegetables.
- Stored in the liver.
- Sufficient reserves present, usually for up to one year.

History

Malnutrition
- Inadequate dietary intake.
- Defective absorption, e.g. steatorrhoea due to hepatobiliary disease.

Eating disorders
- Anorexia.
- Food fads.

Deficiency causes

Symptoms
- Night blindness.
- Dry eyes.
- Scaly skin.

Signs
- White hyperkeratotic patches on the oral mucosa.
- Xerostomia.

Excess of Vitamin A

Symptoms
- Hair loss.
- Bone pain.
- Peeling of the skin.

Signs
- Mucosal atrophy.
- Gingivitis.
- Scaling of the lips.

Vitamin B complex

Vitamin B_1 deficiency
- Causes beri-beri.

Symptoms
- Muscle weakness.
- Burning mouth.

Signs
- Polyneuritis.
- Growth retardation.
- Mental changes.

Vitamin B_2 deficiency

Symptoms
- Sore mouth and tongue.
- Cracked corners of the mouth.

Signs
- Angular cheilitis.
- Glossitis.
- Oral ulceration.
- Patients may also be anaemic.

Vitamin B_6 deficiency

History
- Alcoholism.
- Severe nutritional deficiencies.

Symptoms
- Sore mouth and tongue.

Signs
- Angular cheilitis.
- Glossitis.
- Stomatitis.
- Atrophy of the papillae on the dorsum of the tongue.

Nicotinic acid deficiency

History
- Malnutrition, resulting in pellagra (rough skin).

Symptoms
- Sore mouth and tongue.
- Mouth ulcers.

Signs
- Generalized erythema of oral mucous membrane.
- Atrophy of the tongue papillae.
- Mucosal ulceration may also be seen.
- Ulcers are covered with fibrin.

Vitamin B_{12} deficiency

History
- Inadequate intake, e.g. strict vegetarians (vegans).
- Malabsorption:

1. Pernicious anaemia (failure to produce intrinsic factor), an autoimmune disease.
2. Post-gastrectomy.
3. Crohn's disease.

Symptoms
- Sore tongue, with or without depapillation.
- Neurological symptoms develop in about 10% of patients with pernicious anaemia, e.g. paraesthesia of the extremities which, if untreated, can lead to subacute combined degeneration of the spinal cord.

Diagnostic tests
- Full blood count.
- Serum B_{12} levels.
- Antibodies to parietal cells and/or intrinsic factor.
- Schilling test for B_{12} deficiency.

Vitamin C deficiency (scurvy)

Very rare in the UK.

History
- Inadequate dietary intake.

Symptoms
- Swollen, bleeding gums.
- Loose teeth due to defective collagen production.
- Bone pain.

Signs
- Swelling of gingival margins with ulceration and gingival bleeding.
- Anaemia.
- Mobility of teeth.
- Periodontal bone loss.

N.B. gingival changes, though rare, are similar to those seen in leukaemia.

Diagnostic tests
- Full blood count to exclude blood dyscrasias.
- Specialized haematological investigations, e.g. leukocyte, ascorbic acid concentration.
- Bite-wing or OPT radiograph to determine periodontal bone levels.

Vitamin D deficiency

History
- Dietary deficiency.
- Malabsorption diseases.
- Vitamin D-resistant rickets, an X chromosome-linked disorder of renal phosphate reabsorption.
- Chronic renal failure.
- Pregnancy and lactation.
- Vitamin D deficiency causes surprisingly few oral changes in spite of deformities of the long bones and weight-bearing bones in both rickets and osteomalacia.

Oral symptoms
- Dental pain and swelling caused by pulpitis and dental abscesses can occur in patients with vitamin D-resistant rickets, due to abnormally large pulp chambers with elongated pulp horns.

Signs
- Delayed eruption may occur.
- Abnormal dentine calcification.
- Minimal caries can result in pulpal inflammatory changes.

- Dental radiographs may show increased radiolucency of the jaws and reduced density of the lamina dura surrounding the teeth.

Diagnostic tests
- Haematological investigations.
- Low serum calcium.
- Normal or low serum phosphate.
- Raised alkaline phosphatase levels.

Vitamin E

History
- No relevant history, as there are no specific lesions which develop in humans when vitamin E may be lacking in the diet.
- No oral changes have been recorded in humans with possible vitamin E deficiency.

Vitamin K deficiency

- Required for synthesis of the blood-clotting factors — Prothrombin (II), VII, IX and X.

History
- A defective diet (vitamin K is found in green leafy vegetables).
- Obstructive jaundice.
- Malabsorption syndromes.
- Vitamin K metabolism is impaired by anticoagulant medication, e.g. warfarin, and in severe liver disease.

Symptoms
- As in other bleeding disorders.
- Bleeding gums.
- Prolonged bleeding after surgery, including dental extractions.

Tests
- Haematological investigations.
- There is an increased prothrombin time (PT). Usually expressed as the international normalized ratio (INR); this is of particular importance for patients on oral anticoagulants for whom dental surgery should not be undertaken if the ratio is above 2.5.

2. Endocrine

Pregnancy

History
- Sexually-active woman of child-bearing age who has missed a menstrual period.

Oral symptoms

- Swelling and bleeding of gums (pregnancy gingivitis).
- Discrete gingival swelling (gingival epulis) which bleeds on brushing.

Oral signs

- Generalized marginal gingivitis.
- Gums which bleed on probing.
- Pregnancy epulides present as erythematous gingival swellings (see page 233), usually involving the interdental papilla; they may occur labially and lingually.
- Gingival inflammation which is excessive in view of the patient's oral hygiene levels.
- Occasionally patients with recurrent aphthae may find that their oral ulceration clears completely during pregnancy but in some the ulcers become more severe.

Tests

- Pregnancy tests.
- Radiographs and all drugs should be avoided, whenever possible, particularly during the first trimester.

Pituitary malfunction

Diabetes insipidus

History

- Idiopathic or may be caused by trauma, tumour, vascular disease or infiltration of the pituitary gland, e.g. Hand–Schüller–Christian syndrome.

Symptoms

- Severe thirst.
- Dry mouth.
- Increased frequency of urination.

Signs

- Polydypsia.
- Polyurea (as high as 20 litres per day!).
- Xerostomia.

Growth hormone

History

- Excess growth hormone production gives rise to gigantism if it occurs before the epiphyses fuse or acromegaly in the adult.

- Caused by a pituitary tumour (an adenoma).

Symptoms
- Spacing of teeth and large lower jaw.
- Dentures no longer fit (in acromegaly).

Signs
- Mandibular prognathism.
- Enlargement of nasal and condylar cartilages.
- Scalloping of the lateral margins of the tongue.
- Tongue may enlarge disproportionately.
- Thickening of the skin with accentuation of skin folds.

Tests
- Skull radiographs confirm enlargement of the sella turcica.
- Oral radiographs show hypercementosis and an increase in size of the jaws.
- CT and MRI scan.
- Glucose tolerance tests and growth hormone levels.

Hypopituitarism in children may be caused by a craniopharyngioma or supracellar cyst.

- Growth is depressed, mandibular development retarded and tooth eruption delayed.

Thyroid gland

Hypothyroidism

History
- Congenital hypothyroidism (cretinism).
- In adults (myxoedema).

Oral symptoms in congenital hypothyroidism
- Large lips and tongue.
- Missing teeth.

Oral signs in congenital hypothyroidism
- Enlarged lips and protruding tongue in children.
- Shortening of the base of the skull.
- Flattened bridge of nose.
- Eruption of teeth is delayed.

Oral signs in adults with myxoedema
- Tongue may also be enlarged with scalloped margins, due to indentation by the teeth.

- Loss of hair and thinning of the eyebrows may occur.

Hyperthyroidism (thyrotoxicosis)

Oral signs

- Early eruption of teeth.

Parathyroid glands

Hypoparathyroidism

History

- Thyroid surgery with concurrent removal of parathyroid gland.
- Radiation therapy to thyroid region.
- Idiopathic.

Symptoms

- Discoloured teeth and delayed eruption seen only in the idiopathic form, due to the reduced serum calcium.
- Symptoms of tetany may occur, with numbness and tingling of the arms and legs, together with facial twitching and carpopedal spasms.

Signs

- Delayed eruption.
- Severely mottled teeth due to enamel hypoplasia in the idiopathic form.
- Hypoparathyroidism and chronic mucocutaneous candidiasis (see page 158) are a feature of candidiasis endocrinopathy syndrome.
- Tapping of the facial nerve as it passes over the lower border of the mandible causes facial twitching and facial paraesthesia (Chvostek's sign).
- Carpopedal spasms (Trousseau's sign):
  Occlude the arterial pulse with a sphygmomanometer for 5 minutes. In patients with tetany, spasm of the hands and wrists occurs.
- Radiographs reveal delayed eruption and shortened roots in the idiopathic form.
- In hypoparathyroidism following surgery or radiotherapy there are no abnormal dental findings.

Diagnostic tests

- Reduced serum calcium.
- Raised serum phosphate.

Hyperparathyroidism

History
- Primary — caused by an adenoma or rarely a carcinoma of the parathyroid glands.
- Secondary — due to low serum calcium, the result of renal disease.
- Tertiary — as a result of prolonged secondary disease which then becomes autonomous.

Oral symptoms
- Swellings on gums which are usually painless (epulides).

Oral signs
- Discrete erythematous gingival swellings.
- Adjacent teeth remain vital.

Diagnostic tests
- Biopsy of soft tissue swellings and bony radiolucencies on radiograph confirm a giant cell fibrous lesion, indistinguishable from giant cell granulomas of the jaws.
- Lesions are termed brown tumours or osteitis fibrosa cystica.

Primary and tertiary hyperparathyroidism:
- Serum calcium levels are raised.
- Serum phosphate may be normal or decreased.
- Alkaline phosphatase levels are also normal or increased when there are bony lesions.

Secondary hyperthyroidism:
- Serum calcium levels are normal or decreased.
- Serum phosphate levels are normal or increased in renal failure.
- Alkaline phosphatase levels are normal or increased.

Radiographs
- Loss of lamina dura.
- Some loss of trabeculation and generalized bone rarefaction.
- Giant cell lesions which appear as radiolucencies may be discovered on routine radiological examination.

Pancreas (diabetes mellitus)

History

May be primary
- Juvenile onset (insulin dependent, IDDM).
- Mature onset (non-insulin dependent, NIDDM).

Or secondary to

- Pancreatic damage.
- Endocrine disorders, e.g. acromegaly, Cushing's syndrome and steroid therapy.
- Rare genetic syndromes.

Oral symptoms in the poorly controlled diabetic

- Dry mouth.
- Rarely, tenderness or a burning sensation of the oral mucosa.
- More rapid periodontal breakdown leading to loosening of the teeth and associated pain.
- Gingival swelling due to periodontal abscess formation.

Signs

- Reduced salivary flow.
- Glossitis.
- Oral candidiasis.
- May be increased caries present.
- Advanced periodontal disease.
- Radiographs confirm the extent of carious destruction of the teeth and periodontal bone loss.

Adrenals

Addison's disease

History

Primary hypoadrenocorticism.

Aetiology

- Mainly due to autoimmune disease.
- Adrenal tuberculosis.
- Amyloidosis.
- Neoplasia.
- Histoplasmosis.

Symptoms

- Increase in pigmentation of skin and oral mucosa.

Signs

- Brown or black areas of hyperpigmentation, most commonly on areas exposed to trauma, such as the buccal mucosa at the level of the occlusal plane.
- Also seen on tongue, lips and gingiva.

- No changes seen on radiographs.
- Possible features of chronic mucocutaneous candidiasis.

Cushing's syndrome/disease

History

- Pituitary adenoma causing adrenal hyperplasia.
- Tumours of the adrenal glands.
- Systemic corticosteroid therapy.

Oral signs

- Moon face.
- Candidiasis.

3. Gastrointestinal

Ulcerative colitis

History

- A chronic, inflammatory disease of the mucosa of the large intestine and rectum.
- Affects all age groups.
- More frequently seen in women and young adults.

Oral symptoms

- Recurrent aphthous ulceration, both minor (< 1 cm in diameter) and major (> 1 cm).
- Painful pustules and small ulcers (pyostomatitis vegetans) on the lips, gingiva and palate.
- Rarely isolated ulcers termed pyostomatitis gangrenosum.

Oral signs

- Patients have swollen submandibular lymph glands and are febrile.
- Chronic oral ulceration is seen, in addition to the recurrent oral aphthae and pyostomatitis vegetans described above; these present as irregular ulcers with rolled edges and a grey base.
- Pyostomatitis vegetans appears to be a specific marker of inflammatory bowel disease.
- Oral hairy leukoplakia can occasionally arise in patients treated with long term immunosuppressant therapy.

Diagnostic tests

- Biopsy of oral epithelium in patients with pyostomatitis vegetans confirms the presence of intra-epithelial eosinophilic abscesses.

Crohn's disease

History
- Regional ileitis (Crohn's disease) can involve any part of the gastrointestinal tract but mainly affects the terminal ileum.

Oral symptoms
- Oral ulcers.
- Recurrent or persistent swelling of lips and cheeks.

Oral signs
- Recurrent oral aphthae.
- Diffuse swelling of the cheeks, lips and gingiva.
- Hyperplasia of the mucosa, giving rise to mucosal tags or a cobblestone appearance.
- Linear ulcers which may be large and ragged. Typically seen in the vestibular regions.
- Chronic hyperplastic gingivitis which is erythematous.
- Pyostomatitis vegetans (intra-epithelial abscesses). Rare in Crohn's disease.
- Melkersson–Rosenthal syndrome (facial palsy, facial swelling and fissured tongue).

Diagnostic tests
- Refer to specialist.
- Appropriate gastrointestinal radiology may reveal strictures in the ileum.
- Oral mucosal biopsy may reveal presence of non-caseating granulomas and lymphoedema.
- Colonoscopy or sigmoidoscopy and barium enemas.
- Rectal mucosal biopsy.
- Haematological tests, e.g. serum iron, B_{12} and folate levels may be decreased due to malabsorption.

4. Bone

Paget's disease (osteitis deformans)

History
- A disease of bone where there is disorganization of the normal process of resorption and replacement.
- Present in up to 5% of the population in the UK over the age of 55. Men are affected more frequently than women.
- Aetiology is unknown but a slow virus and other viruses have been suggested as possible causes.

- Many sites may be affected, including the jaws.
- Initially, there is mainly resorption (osteolytic stage).
- This is followed by osteoblastic proliferation (sclerotic stage).

Symptoms

- Bone pain.
- Progressive deafness.
- Deteriorating vision due to optic nerve compression.
- When the jaws are involved, dentures become ill-fitting.

Signs

- Bone deformity, particularly of weight-bearing bones.
- Bossing of frontal bones.
- Symmetrical enlargement of maxilla in malar region (leontiasis ossea).
- In the early stages of the disease when the bone is soft, pathological fracture may occur.
- Enlargement of the jaws, more commonly the maxilla, causes gaps to appear between the teeth.

Diagnostic tests

- Markedly raised serum alkaline phosphatase.
- Calcium or phosphate levels show little or no change.

Radiographs

- Initially, there is radiolucency with loss of lamina dura.
- Root resorption may occur during the osteolytic stage.
- Subsequently, when there is widening of the alveolar ridges, radiographs show a 'cotton wool' appearance of the jaws, together with hypercementosis and pulp calcification.

Complications

- Dental treatment may be complicated during the osteolytic stage by post-extraction haemorrhage.
- In the later stages, extraction is complicated by hypercementosis and chronic osteomyelitis, due to the reduced blood supply to the bone.
- Patients with dentures may have to have regular replacements of their prostheses as the alveolus enlarges.
- Osteosarcoma.
- High-output cardiac failure.

Fibrous dysplasia

History

- Fibro-osseous lesions.
- No relevant medical history.

- Fibrous dysplasia may be monostotic (affecting a single bone) or polyostotic, which is less common (affecting several bones).
- More common in females.
- Most cases involving the jaws are monostotic lesions.
- See also Cherubism, page 261.

Symptoms
- Swellings, due to replacement of the bone with fibrous tissue.
- Jaw lesions usually present in childhood as painless swellings.
- Most will stop enlarging when skeletal growth is complete.
- Patients with polyostotic fibrous dysplasia may also have skin hyperpigmentation (café-au-lait).
- Fibrous dysplasia, skin hyperpigmentation and female precocious puberty is known as Albright's syndrome.

Diagnostic tests
- Serum alkaline phosphatase levels may be raised.
- Calcium and phosphate levels are normal.
- Biopsy and histopathological examination.
- Radiographs show variable appearance — may be ground glass or cystic.

5. Immunologically mediated

Sjögren's syndrome

Introduction.
- Divided into primary Sjögren's syndrome (previously termed Sicca syndrome) with dry mouth and dry eyes, and secondary Sjögren's syndrome where there is dry mouth, dry eyes and rheumatoid arthritis or another connective tissue disease.

History
- No relevant past medical history.
- More than 80% of patients are women with a mean age of onset at 50 years.

Extra-oral symptoms.
- Dry eyes with itching and burning, leading to keratoconjunctivitis sicca.
- Swollen, painful parotid glands.

Oral symptoms
- Dry, sore mouth.
- Difficulty in swallowing, speaking and wearing dentures.
- Dental pain may be present due to increased susceptibility to caries.

Signs
- Dry, erythematous, non-ulcerated mucosa.
- Depapillated, shiny, lobulated tongue.
- Angular cheilitis.
- Oral candidiasis.
- Increased gingival disease.
- Dental caries on cervical and incisal surfaces.
- Salivary glands may, in a minority of cases, develop tender, firm, diffuse, unilateral or bilateral swellings.

Diagnostic tests
- Salivary flow rates.
- Schirmer test shows reduced tear-flow rate.
- Labial salivary gland biopsy shows lymphocytic infiltrate and focal sialadenitis.
- Positive rheumatoid factor.
- Antibodies against extractable nuclear antigens Ro(SS-A) and La(SS-B).
- Haematological examination may reveal a raised ESR and anaemia.
- It is essential for patients to have an ophthalmology examination as the keratoconjunctivitis sicca may be initially asymptomatic but can lead ultimately to impairment or even loss of sight, if untreated.

Radiographs
- Sialography shows sialectasis (typically a 'snowstorm' appearance).
- Salivary scintigraphy with radioactive sodium pertechnetate.

Angio-oedema

Hereditary

History
- Usually transmitted as an autosomal dominant trait.
- Possible family history.
- Due to a deficiency of C1 esterase inhibitor and an abnormality of the complement system.
- May be precipitated by trauma, such as the extraction of a tooth.
- Some attacks follow the injection of drugs including local anaesthesia or emotional stress.
- Previously had a high fatality rate. Can now be prevented by taking the anabolic steriod stanazolol daily and by the administration of C1 esterase inhibitor prior to dental treatment.

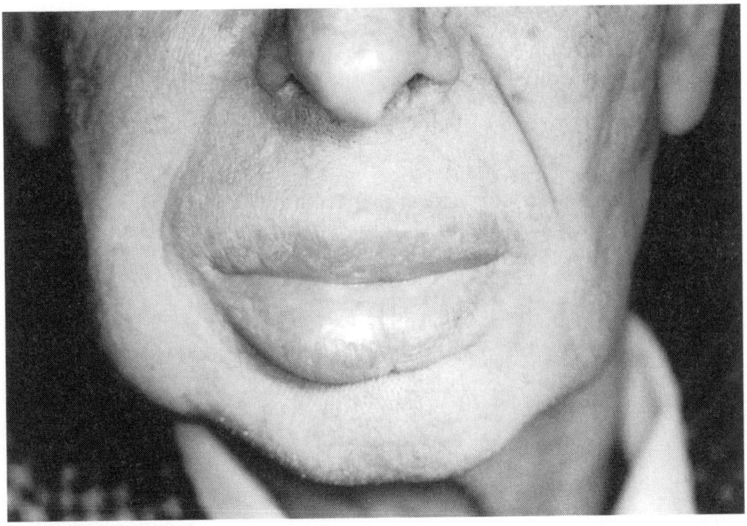

Figure 13.1 Allergic angio-oedema.

Symptoms

- Gastrointestinal upset may precede an attack with abdominal pain, diarrhoea and nausea or vomiting.
- Difficulty in breathing, due to oedema of the glottis.
- Facial swelling.

Allergic angio-oedema (Fig. 13.1)

History

- Previous allergies to drugs or allergens (such as egg protein) in some but not all cases.
- Drugs causing angio-oedema include penicillin and other antibiotics, aspirin and other non-steroidal anti-inflammatory drugs, pimozide and codeine.
- Angio-oedema has also been reported following application of a rubber dam and the use of ethylene imine in 'Scutan'®.
- May be associated with anaphylaxis.

Symptoms

- Swelling of the face, lips and tongue.
- Often there is associated itching.
- Although difficulty in breathing from respiratory obstruction is more common in hereditary angio-oedema, should the swelling spread to the glottis a life-threatening emergency may occur.

Amyloid

History

- A disease in which there is extracellular deposition of an eosinophilic protein material, which has a characteristic fibrillar structure on electron microscopy.

Primary systemic amyloidosis

History

- Rare.
- Males more commonly affected than females.
- The disease usually occurs in patients in their late 60s or early 70s.
- Invariably fatal from renal and cardiac involvement.
- Median survival is only 12 months after diagnosis.

Symptoms

- Pain from oral ulceration.
- Swollen gums and bleeding tendency, due to a deficiency of factors IX and X.
- Dry mouth.

Signs

- Macroglossia (the tongue being firm and may affect speech).
- Gingival swellings.
- Xerostomia.
- Oral petechia.
- Oral ecchymoses.
- Bullae on the tongue which may rupture, leaving ulcers.
- Macular or papular oral lesions

Secondary or reactive amyloidosis

History

- Associated with and secondary to disorders such as rheumatoid arthritis, Crohn's disease and ulcerative colitis.
- Infections, e.g. tuberculosis and bronchietasis.
- Dermatological disease, e.g. psoriasis.
- Neoplasia, e.g. Hodgkin's disease and renal carcinoma.

Clinical features

- May affect many organs, such as the heart, spleen, kidney and adrenal glands.
- Oral signs and symptoms are seen virtually only in the primary type.

- The prognosis for secondary amyloidosis is also poor, with 50% of patients with amyloidosis-complicating rheumatic disease surviving less than 5 years.

Diagnostic tests
- Biopsy, usually rectal.
- Gingival biopsy has been used.
- Serological tests for patients with myeloma-associated amyloid.
- Bone scanning.
- Echocardiography.

Systemic lupus erythematosus

History
- One of the connective tissue diseases.
- More common (eight times) in women than in men and three times more common in negroes than in caucasians.
- An autoimmune disease.
- May also be induced by drugs, such as hydralazine, procainamide, methyldopa, sulphonamides, isoniazid, epanutin and carbamazepine.
- A serious constitutional and multi-system disorder affecting joints, skin, mucous membrane, heart, lungs and kidneys.
- Central nervous system involvement may produce epilepsy and psychoses.
- The production of auto-antibodies may cause thrombocytopenia and haemolytic anaemia.

Symptoms
- The typical picture is of a young woman between the ages of 10 and 40 years with fever, malaise, joint pains and anaemia.
- A facial rash with a 'butterfly' pattern may occur, extending over the bridge of the nose and on to the cheeks.
- Enlargement of the salivary glands, giving rise to secondary Sjögren's syndrome has been reported in up to 30% of cases.

Oral signs
- Keratotic lesions resembling lichen planus are seen in 10–25% of cases.
- The palate is the most common site, although slit-like ulcers may also be seen on the gingival margins.

Diagnostic tests
- Chest radiograph may reveal cardiomegaly or pleural effusion.

Immunological findings
- Hypergammaglobulinaemia.
- Reduced serum complement levels.
- Anti-nuclear antibodies.
- Anti-DNA antibodies.
- Anti-RNA antibodies.
- Rheumatoid factor.
- False-positive serological test for syphilis.

- Antibodies to platelets and other blood cells.
- Biopsies of oral lesions may show epithelial thinning, acanthosis and thickening of the basement membrane.
- There is a diffuse infiltrate of chronic inflammatory cells.
- In addition to anaemia and thrombocytopenia, patients with SLE may also have cardiac disease, renal failure and may be taking corticosteroids and other immunosuppressant drugs.

6. Haematological

Anaemia

Introduction
- May be defined as a reduction in the haemoglobin concentration of the blood below the normal level for the age and gender of the patient.
- Normal range: male 13.0–18.0 g/dl, female 11.5–16.5 g/100 ml.

Causes
- Blood loss, e.g. menorrhagia, trauma, blood loss from the gastrointestinal tract due to an ulcer or carcinoma and bleeding from the genito-urinary tract.
- Excessive destruction — haemolytic anaemias, e.g. sickle-cell anaemia and thalassaemia.
- Impaired absorption, e.g. vitamin B_{12} (absorption depends on intrinsic factor produced by the gastric mucosa).
- Malabsorption also occurs in coeliac disease, Crohn's disease, following gastrectomy (B_{12}) and other malabsorption states.
- Increased demand for haematinics — pregnancy.
- Poor intake of haematinics — Fe, B_{12}, folic acid (poverty, alcoholism, food fads).
- Aplastic anaemia and leukaemias.
- Drug associated, e.g. alcohol, barbiturates, methotrexate and phenytoin, can cause folic acid deficiencies.

General symptoms
- May be symptom-free.
- Can tire easily.
- Shortness of breath on exertion.
- Tingling of the extremities.
- Light-headedness.
- Faintness.
- Chest pain (angina) on exertion.
- Brittle nails with koilonychia (spoon-shaped) and lustreless fingernails.
- Pallor.
- Patients with sickle-cell anaemia suffer with painful crises caused by clumping of the erythrocytes, as they deform into the sickle shape when deoxygenated; symptoms include bone pain, due to blockage of minor blood vessels; there may be organ infarcts affecting the lungs and spleen.
- Oral signs and symptoms particularly prominent in the deficiency anaemias.

Oral symptoms
- Sore tongue.
- Painful tongue.
- Sore mouth.
- Difficulty swallowing (Paterson–Kelly/Plummer–Vinson syndrome).

Oral signs
- Atrophic glossitis — smooth, inflamed tongue.
- Angular cheilitis — more common in folate and iron-deficiency than pernicious anaemia.
- Oral ulceration.
- Oral candidiasis may be a feature of chronic mucocutaneous candidiasis and iron deficiency (familial type).
- Glossitis and stomatitis are marked in B_{12} deficiency and may present as a tender, raw, oedematous and atrophic tongue.
- Paterson–Kelly/Plummer–Vinson syndrome, i.e. dysphagia and glossitis together with an iron deficiency anaemia is associated with a much increased risk of post-cricoid carcinoma.
- Pallor — N.B. the oral mucosal colour is a more sensitive sign, as are the nail beds and the conjunctivae than skin colour in the anaemic patient.

Diagnostic tests

Iron deficiency
- Full blood count to show haemoglobin levels, red blood cell values, mean corpuscular volume and mean corpuscular haemoglobin concentration.

- Packed cell volume (haematocrit).
- Serum ferritin and serum iron levels are reduced in iron deficiency anaemia and the total iron binding capacity is raised.

Vitamin B_{12} deficiency
- Vitamin B_{12} is a megaloblastic anaemia.
- The cells are macrocytic.
- There is a low serum B_{12} and a positive Schilling test.

Folate deficiency
- Folate deficiency also causes a megaloblastic anaemia with macrocytosis.
- Red cell folate values are low.

Sickle-cell anaemia
- Can be confirmed by haemoglobin electrophoresis.
- Other special investigations may also be required.

Thalassaemia.
- A hypochromic microcytic anaemia with increased red blood cell fragility and haemolysis.
- In thalassaemia, serum iron and ferritin levels are normal or raised and the total iron-binding capacity is normal.
- There is an increase, however, in HbF, the foetal haemoglobin.

Radiological changes

Sickle-cell anaemia
- Thickening of the skull and a 'hair on end' pattern to the trabeculae.
- There may be bony radiolucencies as a result of infarction in the mandible or due to osteomyelitis.
- Bone marrow hyperplasia may result in rarefaction of the mandibular bone and apparent osteoporosis.

Thalassaemia
- The alveolar bone rarefaction produces a 'chicken wire' appearance.
- There may also be spacing of the teeth and drifting of incisors.

Note. General anaesthesia is hazardous in patients with anaemia and, wherever possible, the underlying cause should be treated before general anaesthesia is carried out.

Jaundice

Introduction

- Jaundice is not a disease in itself but is a clinical manifestation of a number of diseases which result in a breakdown in the metabolism and excretion of bilirubin. This leads to an accumulation of bilirubin in the blood and tissues.

Causes

- Obstructive, such as gallstones and carcinoma of the pancreas.
- Haemolytic anaemias, such as sickle-cell disease, thalassaemia, hereditary spherocytosis, malaria, glucose-6-phosphate dehydrogenase deficiency, neonatal jaundice.
- Infections such as viral hepatitis (e.g. hepatitis A, hepatitis B or hepatitis C viruses).
- Congenital disorders, such as Gilbert's syndrome and Dubin–Johnson syndrome.
- Hepatic cirrhosis and primary biliary cirrhosis.

Systemic symptoms

- Nausea.
- Vomiting.
- Loss of appetite.
- Itching.
- Yellow discoloration of skin and eyes.

Signs

- Yellow discoloration of the skin, oral mucosa and sclera.
- Abdominal tenderness.
- In neonatal jaundice hyperbilirubinaemia may cause green discoloration and pigmentation of tooth dentine and enamel hypoplasia.

Diagnostic tests

Serological tests for markers in patients with suspected hepatitis B or history of hepatitis B must include:

- Hepatitis B surface antigen. Positive in carriers and in acute infection.
- Hepatitis B e-antigen and e-antibody. Presence of the e-antigen occurs only in those who are also surface antigen positive and indicates high infectivity.

E-antibody presence and loss of e-antigen in the serum indicates recovery. N.B. Patients with surface antigen may also have e-antibody. This still indicates a carrier state but a lower infective risk than those patients with both surface antigen and e-antigen in their serum.

Note:

- Core antibodies to hepatitis B may be also detected in the serum of patients exposed to hepatitis B.
- Hepatitis B surface antibody will be present in the serum of patients who have immunity, either through infection and recovery or through vaccination.
- Hepatitis C antibody markers are seen in patients who have been exposed to hepatitis C virus. As with HIV, these are not considered neutralizing or protective antibodies.
- Patients with jaundice may have bleeding tendencies and therefore blood samples are required to test for an increased prothrombin time (PT).
- The activated partial thromboplastin time (APTT) may also be prolonged.
- Bleeding from oesophageal varices may cause anaemia.
- Specific enzymes, e.g. aspartate transaminase (AST) and aniline transaminase (ALT) are amongst those which have raised serum levels in liver disease.

Leukaemia

Introduction

- Leukaemias are diseases caused by neoplastic proliferation of cells which form white blood cells within the bone marrow.
- They occur in acute and chronic forms.
- The clinical signs and symptoms of leukaemias are those of anaemia, infection, bleeding, oral ulceration and lymphadenopathy.

Acute leukaemias

Acute lymphoblastic leukaemia (ALL)

- The commonest malignancy in childhood.
- Peak incidence between 2 and 10 years.

Acute myeloblastic leukaemia (Fig. 13.2)

- The most common acute leukaemia seen in adults.

Systemic symptoms

- Weakness.
- Loss of appetite.
- Bleeding.

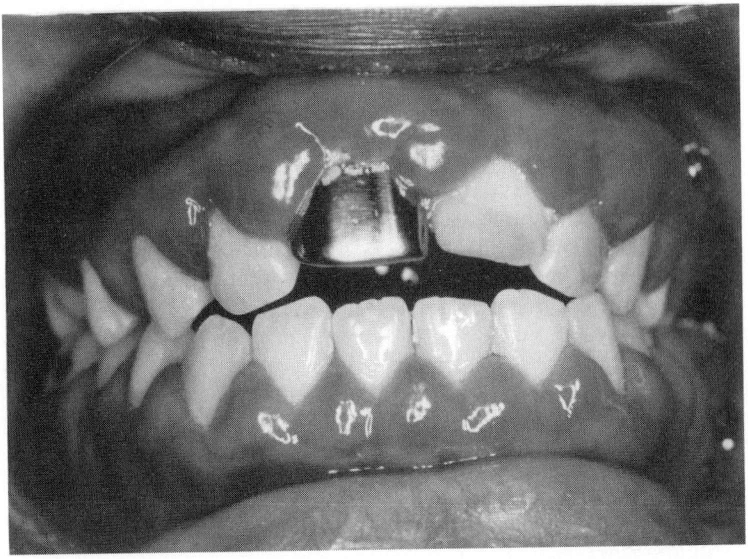

Figure 13.2 Swollen gingivae of acute myeloblastic leukaemia.

- Bone pain.
- Weight loss.
- Bruising.

Systemic signs
- Pyrexia.
- Splenomegaly.
- Pallor.
- Infections.
- Purpura (skin rash due to bleeding from capillaries – individual purple spots known as petechiae).
- Lymphadenopathy.

Oral symptoms
- Swollen, bleeding gums.
- Painful ulcers.
- Painful enlarged glands in neck.

Oral signs
- Oral manifestations may be the initial complaint and can be present in up to 90% of cases.
- Gingival swelling.
- Petechia.
- Oral ecchymosis (bruising).

- Mucosal or gingival ulceration.
- Haemorrhage.
- Mucosal pallor.
- Fungal and herpetic infections are common.
- Infective organisms include candida, aspergillus, pseudomonas and klebsiella.
- Acute myeloblastic leukaemia is particularly associated with gingival swelling and many of the drugs used in treatment of leukaemia can cause oral side effects such as dry mouth and candidiasis.
- Radiological examination may show thinning of the lamina dura and loss of alveolar bone.
- Roots of developing teeth may also be affected.

Diagnostic tests
- Full blood count should be requested for all patients with unexplained gingival swelling, cervical lymphadenopathy and oral ulceration.
- Microbiological culture and sensitivity tests are required for oral infections in order that the appropriate antimicrobial treatment is prescribed.

Chronic leukaemias

Chronic lymphocytic leukaemia
- The most common chronic leukaemia.
- Usually affects men over the age of 60 years.
- Anaemia and thrombocytopenia can occur.

Systemic symptoms
- Fever.
- Weight loss.
- Loss of appetite.
- Bleeding gums.
- Infections.
- Swollen glands.

Signs
- Enlarged lymph nodes.
- Splenomegaly and hepatomegaly.
- Skin infiltration by leukaemic cells may occur.
- Gingival swelling less common than in acute leukaemias.
- Gingival haemorrhage, oral petechia and oral ulceration.
- Herpes simplex, zoster and candidal infections may be present.

Diagnostic tests
- Full blood count essential.

Chronic myeloid leukaemia (CML)
- Accounts for 20% of all leukaemias.
- Peak incidence between 40–60 years of age.
- Enlargement of spleen and liver are common.
- Can eventually transform to an acute phase with anaemia, bleeding and infection.
- Weight loss and joint pains may also occur.
- In CML, leukaemic infiltration of lacrimal and salivary glands can cause Mikulicz's syndrome (enlargement of glands with dry mouth and dry eyes – also seen in patients with lymphoma, sarcoidosis and tuberculosis).
- Dental and oral treatment for patients with leukaemia should only be undertaken after full consultation with the patient's physician.

Thrombocytopenia

History
- Idiopathic thrombocytopenic purpura.
- Leukaemia.
- Aplastic anaemia.
- Systemic lupus erythematosus.
- AIDS/HIV.
- Normal platelet count 150–400 $\times$ 10^9/l.
- Thrombocytopenia occurs when levels fall below 100 $\times$ 10^9/l.

Symptoms
- Bruise easily.
- Tendency to postoperative bleeding.

Signs
- Purpura and ecchymosis on skin.
- Intraoral petechiae.
- Spontaneous gingival bleeding.

Diagnostic tests
- Full blood count.

Further reading

Jones, J.H. and Mason, D.K. (1990) *Oral Manifestations of Systemic Disease*, 2nd edn. London: Ballière-Tindall.

Scully, C. and Cawson, R.A. (1998) *Medical Problems in Dentistry*, 4th edn. Oxford: Wright.

14

Oral consequences of medication

Summary

Introduction

Medication may be:

- Prescription
- Non-prescription

Medical history

Dental history

Effects may be:

- Negative
- Masking
- Suppressive
- Positive

Oral consequences of medication

1. Local effects
   - Allergy – flavouring agents
   - Alteration of oral flora – topical antibiotics, steroids
   - Caries – sugary cough mixtures
   - Chemical irritation – aspirin, oil of cloves
   - Delayed healing – topical steroids
   - Erosion – acidic liquid medicines
   - Extrinsic tooth discoloration – chlorhexidine
2. Systemic effects
   - Allergy
     - Angio-oedema
     - Erythema multiforme
     - Exfoliative stomatitis
     - Fixed drug eruption
     - Lichenoid reaction
   - Bad breath (halitosis) – disulfiram
   - Cervical lymphadenopathy – phenytoin
   - Delayed healing – systemic steroids
   - Depression of immune system – fungal and viral mucosal infection
   - Depression of bone marrow – oral ulceration, purpura, gingival bleeding
   - Facial muscle tics – phenothiazines

continued

Facial pain – phenothiazines
Gingival hyperplasia – phenytoin
Hypersecretion of saliva – clozapine
Intrinsic tooth discoloration – tetracycline, fluoride
Lupoid reaction – procainamide
Oral pigmentation – phenothiazines, heavy metal poisoning
Pemphigus/pemphigoid-like reactions – penicillamine
Salivary gland pain – antihypertensives
Salivary gland swelling – phenothiazine, sulphonamide
Taste perception alteration – metronidazole, ACE inhibitors.
Trigeminal paraesthesia – acetazolamide
Xerostomia (dry mouth) – tricyclic antidepressants, etc

Reporting suspected adverse drug reactions

Introduction

Medication may be obtained by prescription or 'over-the-counter' (e.g. aspirin). In addition, the 'recreational' abuse of illegally obtained substances is widespread.

The medical history

- Should include a list of all tablets, medicines, pills, etc (see Chapter 2).
- May include details of medical conditions that may suggest possible use of medication; a history of epilepsy, for example, may suggest possible use of phenytoin, while a history of asthma may suggest possible use of a steroid inhaler.

While a patient is unlikely to be deliberately misleading about their medication, the history may be incomplete as a result of:

- Confusion, particularly the elderly.
- Self-medication with non-prescription drugs may not be considered (by the patient) to be relevant.
- A patient may be reluctant to admit to medication and the underlying problem, e.g. antibiotics for a sexually transmitted disease or use of antidepressants.
- A patient may be reluctant to admit to self-medication, particularly drug abuse.

- Names and dosages of most prescription medications are difficult to remember.
- Neither the prescriber nor the manufacturer knows the full action of a drug; drug interactions and idiosyncratic reactions may occur.
- When many prescription medicines are taken, one or more may be forgotten.

If the type or dosage of any medication is in doubt, ask the patient to bring the medication and any packaging and advice sheets to the next appointment. If any difficulties remain, the patient's medical practitioner should be contacted.

The dental history

- May include details of dental problems that may suggest the possible use of medicaments; recent toothache may have been self-treated using oil of cloves or an aspirin placed in the buccal sulcus; a gingivitis/periodontitis may have been treated by use of a chlorhexidine mouth rinse.
- Some oral changes are characteristic of certain medications, e.g. tetracycline staining of teeth, gingival hyperplasia with phenytoin.

Oral consequences of medication may be due to a local action in the mouth or to a systemic effect. The effects are usually negative (e.g. aspirin burn) but may be masking, suppressive and (occasionally) positive:

Masking

- Medication masks (conceals) the symptoms of oral disease, e.g. silent progression of an oral infection when inflammation is masked by use of steroids.

Suppression

- Medication taken for another condition may suppress the progress of a dental disease, e.g. antibiotics may suppress (but not cure) a dental abscess.

Positive effect

- Medication taken for another condition cures an oral disease; the value of metronidazole in the treatment of acute necrotizing ulcerative gingivitis was recognized in this way.

Oral consequences of medication

1. Local effects

i. Allergy

- Local allergic reactions may (rarely) be seen following use of flavouring agents.
- Lichenoid reactions, which can be clinically indistinguishable from the white patches of oral lichen planus, may occur with oral antidiabetics (for example).

ii. Alteration of oral flora

- Thrush and other types of candidiasis complicate oral treatment with antibiotics (especially tetracycline).
- Oropharyngeal thrush is an occasional side-effect of corticosteroid inhalers.
- Resistant organisms may colonize the oral cavity as a result of prolonged antibiotic use.

iii. Caries

- Some medications, particularly cough mixtures and lozenges, contain sugar in an attempt to improve flavour and acceptability to children.
- Prolonged use of sugar-containing medications may lead to rampant caries.

iv. Chemical irritation

- Aspirin tablets allowed to dissolve in the sulcus in an (erroneous) attempt to self-treat toothache can lead to a white patch followed by ulceration.
- Choline salicylate gels and potassium chloride tablets are also irritant to the mucosa.
- Flavouring agents, particularly essential oils, may cause contact hypersensitivity of the skin. While mucosal involvement is uncommon, cinnamon in toothpaste has been implicated.
- Eugenol (oil of cloves) placed in a painful carious dental cavity is an age-old remedy; if the eugenol spills onto the mucosa, a burn may be produced.

v. Delayed healing

- Delayed healing of trauma or surgical sites may result from use of topical steroids.

vi. Erosion of teeth

- Some medications, in liquid form, are acidic (e.g. saliva substitutes designed for the edentulous, carbolic acid-containing mouthwashes).
- Prolonged use of acidic medications by the dentate may lead to severe acid erosion of teeth.

vii. Extrinsic tooth discoloration

- Brown staining of the teeth follows the use of a chlorhexidine mouthwash, spray or gel, but can be removed by polishing.
- Ferric salts in liquid form can stain surface enamel black.

2. Systemic effects

i. Allergy

Angio-oedema

- Acute allergic angio-oedema is characterized by rapid development of an oedematous swelling, e.g. periorbital.
- If the larynx is involved, resulting respiratory obstruction may be fatal.
- May occur alone or in association with anaphylactic shock.
- Aspirin, penicillin and ACE inhibitors have been implicated but minute amounts of many allergens may induce the change in the susceptible.

Erythema multiforme

- May follow the use of drugs, including penicillin, phenytoin, chlorpropamide and phenobarbitone.
- However, a positive history of drug use is not always present.
- The lips are swollen, crusted and bleeding and the oral mucosa is extensively ulcerated.
- Characteristic 'target'-shaped lesions may be seen on the skin; these are large (1 cm diameter) red macules with a cyanotic centre (superficially similar to an archery target, hence the name).
- A severe conjunctivitis may accompany these lesions.

Exfoliative stomatitis and dermatitis

- Are seen as widespread erosions of oral mucosa and skin due to destruction of the epithelium.
- These are severe and dangerous drug reactions and can be fatal.
- Gold, phenylbutazone and barbiturates have been implicated.

Fixed drug eruptions

- Are characterized by sharply circumscribed skin lesions occur-

ring in the same place each time a particular drug (e.g. phenolphthalein) is taken.
- Involvement of the oral mucosa is rare.

Lichenoid reaction
- Can be clinically indistinguishable from the white patches of oral lichen planus (see Chapter 11).
- Drugs associated with the appearance of white striae and plaques, atrophic changes and ulceration include NSAIDs, methyldopa, metronidazole, chloroquine, oral antidiabetics, diuretics, phenothiazines and gold.

ii. Bad breath (halitosis)
- Is most commonly due to habits (smoking, alcohol) or oral sepsis (especially periodontal disease).
- May also be caused by dry mouth or systemic disease:
  Airway infections
  Liver disease
  Kidney disease
  Gastrointestinal disease
  Diabetic ketosis
- Drugs causing halitosis include disulfiram, chloral hydrate and dimethyl sulphoxide.
- May be delusional when associated with depression, hypochondria or other psychogenic disorder.

iii. Cervical lymphadenopathy
- Has been noted with phenytoin and phenylbutazone.

iv. Delayed healing
- Delayed healing of trauma and surgical sites may be a consequence of systemic steroid use.

v. Depression of the immune system
- Immunosuppression, for example following organ transplantation, may allow fungal (candidal) and viral (often herpetic) mucosal infections, induce gingival bleeding and allow a deterioration in pre-existing periodontal disease.

vi. Depression of bone marrow

Defective white cell production
- If severe may lead to agranulocytosis with necrotizing ulceration of the gingivae and throat.

- Oral ulceration commonly occurs in patients treated with cytotoxic drugs, especially methotrexate, and gold, penicillamine, captopril and other ACE inhibitors.

Defective red cell production

- Folate deficiency and macrocytic anaemia is an occasional complication of long-term phenytoin treatment.
- Oral changes may include severe aphthous ulceration.

Defective haemostasis

- Thrombocytopenia may be drug related (including the above) and may cause bleeding at the gingival margins, which may be spontaneous or may follow mild trauma.

vii. Facial muscle tics

- Involuntary movements of the muscles of facial expression have been recorded following use of a number of drugs, including phenothiazines, phenytoin and carbamazepine.

viii. Facial pain (see also Chapters 5 and 6)

- May occasionally be caused by drugs such as phenothiazines.

ix. Gingival hyperplasia

- Hyperplasia of the gingivae is a common side-effect of phenytoin and sometimes of cyclosporin or nifedipine (and some other calcium-channel blockers).
- The degree of hyperplasia varies, but particularly involves the interdental papillae.
- The hyperplasia is plaque related and can be controlled by efficient plaque removal.

x. Hypersecretion of saliva

- Some drugs (e.g. clozapine) can increase saliva production.
- This is not a problem unless the patient has difficulty swallowing.
- However, some patients experience problems with dribbling of excess saliva and may develop angular cheilitis.

xi. Intrinsic tooth discoloration

Tetracycline staining

- Intrinsic staining of the teeth is most commonly caused by tetracyclines.
- They will affect the teeth if given at any time from the fourth month *in utero* until the age of 12 years.

- All tetracyclines are implicated and the colour depends on the tetracycline used, varying from yellow to grey.
- The teeth involved, position and width of the band of discoloration indicate the age at which the tetracycline was taken and the duration.

Fluorosis
- Excessive ingestion of fluoride during tooth development leads to dental fluorosis with mottling (white and/or brown) of the enamel and areas of hypoplasia or pitting.

xii. Lupoid reaction
- A systemic lupus erythematosus (SLE)-like reaction (see page 281) may be precipitated by drugs including hydralazine and procainamide.

xiii. Oral pigmentation
- Discoloration is caused by deposition of heavy metals, such as lead or mercury, in the gingival tissues. This is rarely seen nowadays.
- Phenothiazines have been reported to induce oral pigmentation.
- Prolonged use of topical antibiotics and antiseptic mouthrinses may cause dark (even black) discoloration of the dorsum of the tongue, possibly as a result of overgrowth of pigment-forming organisms ('black hairy tongue').

xiv. Pemphigus/pemphigoid-like reactions
- In a small minority of cases, the vesicles, bullae and resulting ulcers of pemphigus vulgaris and mucous membrane pemphigoid (see pages 202–204) may be initiated by drugs, including penicillamine.

xv. Salivary gland pain
- Pain in the salivary glands has been reported with some antihypertensives (e.g. bethanidine, clonidine, methyldopa) and with vinca alkaloids.

xvi. Swelling of salivary glands
- Swelling of the salivary glands may occur with iodides, antithyroid drugs, phenothiazines, and sulphonamides.

xvii. Taste perception alteration
- Many drugs affect taste perception, including penicillamine,

griseofulvin, captopril (and other ACE inhibitors), carbimazole and metronidazole.

xviii. Trigeminal paraesthesia

- Has been reported to be consequent to use of a wide variety of drugs but particularly acetazolamide.

xix. Xerostomia (dry mouth)

- The most common effect that drugs have on the salivary glands is to reduce salivary flow.
- Patients with a dry mouth may develop burning, fragile mucosa and may have poor oral hygiene as a result.
- They may develop rampant dental caries, periodontal disease, intolerance of dentures, and oral infections (especially candidiasis).
- Many drugs may cause xerostomia, but particularly tricyclic antidepressants.
- In view of the widespread (and increasing) use of tricyclic antidepressants and the serious dental consequences, this is an important adverse reaction.
- Excessive use of diuretics can also result in xerostomia.

Reporting suspected adverse drug reactions

- The Committee on Safety of Medicines 'yellow card' is used to report suspected adverse drug reactions.
- Where the reaction follows use of a recently introduced product, the requirement is to report all suspected reactions.
- The card also requires a record of all other drugs taken in the previous 3 months, including self-medication.
- Where the suspected reaction occurs with an established product, the requirement is to report serious or unusual reactions, but not minor reactions.

Further reading

Dental Practitioners' Formulary and British National Formulary. Royal Pharmaceutical Society of Great Britain.

Scully, C. and Cawson, R.A. (1998) *Medical Problems in Dentistry*, 4th edn. Oxford: Wright.

Index

Page numbers printed in **bold** type refer to figures.